Collaboration

in Nursing

Contributors

Joyce Patricia Brockhaus
Linda S. Cape
Doris Asselmeier England
Audrey Kalafatich
Amy Hemme Kennedy
Carol Hill Luckey
Bobbie J. Mackay
Robin Moushey
Mary Mills Redman
Anne T. Richardson
Valann Tasch

Collaboration
in Nursing

Edited by
Doris Asselmeier England, RN, MSN, FAAN
Children's Hospital at Washington University Medical Center
St. Louis, Missouri

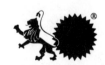

AN ASPEN PUBLICATION®
Aspen Systems Corporation
Rockville, Maryland
Royal Tunbridge Wells
1986

Library of Congress Cataloging in Publication Data
Main entry under title:

Collaboration in nursing.

"An Aspen publication."
Includes bibliographies and index.
1. Nursing—Social aspects. 2. Medical cooperation. 3. Team nursing. I. England, Doris
Asselmeier. [DNLM: 1. Interprofessional Relations. 2. Nursing—trends. 3. Patient. Care
Team. WX 162.5 C697]
RT86.5.C65   1985   610.73   85-18640
ISBN: 0-87189-247-2

Editorial Services: Carolyn Ormes

Library of Congress Catalog Card Number: 85-18640
ISBN: 0-87189-247-2

Printed in the United States of America

1 2 3 4 5

This book is dedicated to the staff of St. Louis Children's Hospital for their caring and support and to T.R.S. for his inspiration and encouragement.

Table of Contents

Foreword

Throughout nursing's history, interest has been expressed in the development of collaborative relationships between physicians and nurses. In more contemporary times, collaboration between doctors and nurses is strongly supported through various professional organizations as well as through the practice of individual care providers. In the early and mid 1960s, the American Nurses' Association and the American Medical Association held national conferences to examine the concept of collaboration and colleagueship, and in 1971, the National Joint Practice Commission (NJPC) was established for the purpose of "nurses and physicians collaborating as colleagues to provide care." In 1983, the report of the National Commission on Nursing (NCN), an independent commission sponsored by the American Hospital Association, the Hospital Research and Education Trust Fund, and the American Hospital Supply Corporation identified effective nurse-physician relationships as critical for the health care field. The need for these two primary providers—doctor and nurse—to work together was recognized with the establishment by the NCN of the goal for hospital organizational structures to be developed in a manner that would facilitate nurse-physician collaboration.

Thus, collaboration is a behavior valued not only in nursing but also by others in the health field and is frequently spoken of as a need or an activity to be accomplished. Unfortunately, collaboration is often viewed in very narrow ways; the nurse practitioner and primary care physician in "collaborative practice" or a joint practice team within the hospital establishing protocols for "collaborative practice" or single episode conflict resolution activities being viewed as "collaborative practice." All of these encompass the essential element of "working together" described by the authors of this book as fundamental to collaboration, but, as pointed out by Doris England and her colleagues, in no way can collaboration in today's health care system be considered from such a limited view. Collaboration is a high-level behavior specific to the professional role and should be an expectation between all professionals. The need to develop practice systems that allow professionals to have time for planning and communication is essential. Time is necessary in order to develop the respect and trust required for mutual sharing and goal setting, outcomes expected in all collaborative activities.

The authors have successfully expanded some common notions of collaboration. They appropriately suggest that the skills of collaboration are applicable in all of nursing's relationships, including the client–nurse relationship. They provide a good foundation for applying the principles of collaborative practice broadly and are pragmatic in their approach to the underlying theories. This book is an excellent contribution to the field and should be useful for all nurse professionals whether their area of practice is predominantly nursing service or nursing education.

Joyce C. Clifford, R.N., F.A.A.N.
Vice President, Nursing and Nurse-in-Chief
Beth Israel Hospital
Boston, Massachusetts

Preface

High technology, rapid advances, specialization, and dwindling dollars for health care have forced rapid and sometimes painful changes in health care institutions. The need for open communication, coordination, and decision making among professionals has become a must. Inefficiency and duplication of effort can no longer be afforded in increasingly competitive and cost conscious health care delivery systems. The intent of this book is to describe the "what," the "why," and the "how" of all facets of collaboration in nursing to improve efficiency, productivity, and professional accountability and satisfaction.

Collaborative practice is more than one physician and one nurse taking care of a group of patients. A definition of physician-nurse collaboration is stated in the *Summary Report and Recommendations* of the National Commission on Nursing, April 1983.

> A jointly determined relationship between the nurses and physicians working together in practice. The purpose of the practice is to integrate their care regimen into a single comprehensive approach to their patients' needs. The practitioners themselves define their roles in consonance with state laws, professional practice acts, policies of the hospital, and the special clinical needs of their particular fields.[1]

Yet the scope of professional collaborative practice extends beyond this definition and physician-nurse collaborative practice. Therefore, this book will be theory-based but will also describe *how* professional collaborative practice is accomplished, *why* it is successful, *what* it does for professionals, and *what* it contributes to health care institutions, but most of all *how* it contributes to patient welfare and recovery and therefore cost savings. We believe that patient outcome is enhanced by professionals working together

xiii

with others as opposed to professionals working toward autonomy. We believe this book will make it apparent that collaboration contributes significantly not only to patient outcome but to cost savings.

Collaborative practice is not just an idea or an abstract concept. It has been operational at St. Louis Children's Hospital for ten years. It may be of interest to the readers that the process of putting this book together was a collaborative effort. Each author discussed her outline and subsequent drafts in group sessions to elicit constructive criticism and to avoid unnecessary duplication.

Although the chapters are written by the St. Louis Children's Hospital clinical nurse specialists and myself, there are contributions from physicians, nurse managers, and administrators via interview.

The primary target populations for the book are persons who practice and/ or teach at the graduate level in nursing, health care administration, and other health care professions. However, all who are interested in developing team concepts including, but not limited to, administrators, health educators, physicians, and so on, can benefit from the content of this book. Even though the book was written by hospital-based practitioners, the principles and practices of collaboration are applicable to all settings where nursing plays a major role.

Doris A. England, R.N., M.S.N., F.A.A.N.
Editor

NOTE

1. National Commission on Nursing, *Summary Report and Recommendations* (Chicago, Ill.: National Commission on Nursing, 1983), p. 37.

Part I

Chapter 1

Collaboration: A Strategy for Now and the Future—A Nurse Executive's Viewpoint

Doris Asselmeier England, R.N., M.S.N., F.A.A.N.

What collaborative relationships are important to successful nursing organizations within successful institutions? How do collaborative strategies contribute to patient outcome? What contribution does collaborative practice make to containing and controlling costs?

This and following chapters address these questions and illustrate that utilizing the full potential of *all* health care team members, reducing duplication of effort, minimizing confrontation, enhancing patients' participation in care, and increasing patient/client compliance will contribute significantly to the two primary goals of collaborative practice—improved patient outcome and cost reduction.

A discussion of structure and basic management philosophies, or the framework within which collaborative practice takes place, will set the stage for subsequent discussions.

To evaluate how structure affects positively the work of the nurse delivering patient care, one must look at the level of the organization where decision making takes place and at which support systems are in place to support those decisions. Structure also raises the issues of trust and span of control. Both concepts are interrelated and important to the overall discussion of collaborative practice models.

THE VALUE OF A DECENTRALIZED STRUCTURE

The organizational charts of a decentralized structure can be viewed from several perspectives (see Figure 1-1). Not only does the first chart run off the page and make people gasp for breath, but it also causes them to scream, "Too much span of control."

The second chart is not only neater and helps people breathe easier (which is not the purpose), it is the way a decentralized system can work. It

3

Figure 1-1 Decentralized Organizational Charts

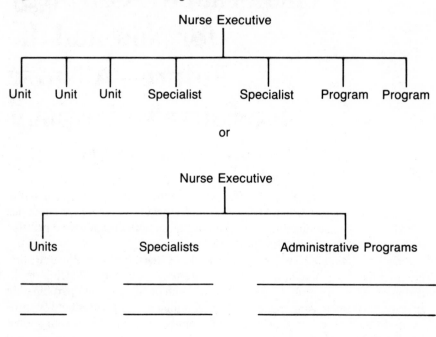

shows a formal and informal mechanism for grouping similar areas and functions and provides an opportunity for the peer-designated leader or emerging leader of the peer group to set the pace and, more importantly, to facilitate decision making within the group.

In a decentralized system certain decisions are delegated to the staff nurse because the philosophy basic to a decentralized system is: the quality of the decision improves in relationship to the closeness of the decision maker to the problem to be solved. Therefore, if the patient is the source of the problem to be solved, then the primary nurse as the direct care deliverer is more likely to make a quality decision than is the head nurse, supervisor, and most certainly the nurse executive. This will be discussed in depth in subsequent chapters. The fallacy or danger in that philosophy is when the decision is contrary to hospital or department philosophy. However, if the design of the philosophy was a collaborative effort within the department, the risk of that situation occurring is unlikely.

Decentralization also raises the issues of trust and span of control. There really is no definitive number of persons in a line relationship that is "ideal" or "good." Most organizational theorists, however, would say that more than six is too many. It is my firm belief that it is not the specific number of persons reporting in the line that makes an organization good or ideal, it is the scope of responsibility and the *who* and *how* of the organization. The "who" must be well-prepared, self-disciplined nurse managers. The "how" must include a trust relationship. For example, when a trust relationship exists between manager and staff, it is not necessary to have daily or even weekly reporting. It is assumed by both parties that programs are proceeding as scheduled and problems are being solved to the benefit of all. Only exceptions and nonresolutions are reported.

MISSION AND POLICY

In addition to a trust relationship up and down the line and across lines, nursing's ability to interface with the entire institution depends on the nurse executive and his or her organizational relationship to the board, administration, medical staff, and nursing staff. As a member of executive management, the nurse executive is in tune with the institution's policy and planning activity and is therefore in a position to share pertinent information with the various staff groups.

Let's take a look at the mission statement of an organization. This is (or should be) where major organizational direction is derived.

A comprehensive mission statement tells you what you believe, gives you consistency of purpose, and becomes the framework for all your hospital policy formulation. It is your source of direction, your reason for being, and it acknowledges all your community relationships.[1]

Following are two mission statements. At first reading they may seem very similar, but a closer review reveals important differences.

Mission statement 1:

Hospital X is a not-for-profit, charitable institution dedicated to excellence of patient care, education, and research. We offer health services to all persons in need, regardless of race, creed, color, religion, sex, national origin, handicap, or ability to pay.

Mission statement 2:

Hospital Y is a not-for-profit, charitable institution dedicated to excellence of patient care. The interrelationship of patient care, education, and research is essential to that excellence. We offer health services to all persons in need, regardless of race, creed, color, religion, sex, national origin, or handicap. We seek to make our services accessible to the community at a reasonable cost. We operate the hospital in ways that will ensure financial viability.

Obviously these are not complete mission statements, but they illustrate the point that the mission sets direction and thus sets the stage for collaboration. What are the subtle differences in these two mission statements? How do the differences in these two statements influence nursing's ability to interface collaboratively with all levels of the organization and all health care members?

Following is a description of a situation and a demonstration of the flow of decision making within the boundaries of each of the mission statements presented.

Mr. Jones entered the emergency room with multiple injuries that resulted from an automobile accident. Certain fractures were evident, but the extent of the internal injuries was unknown.

If this scenario had taken place in Hospital X (mission statement 1), the nurse's response and followthrough would probably complete the scenario as follows:

The physician was called. X-rays and laboratory tests and other diagnostic tests were ordered. While the patient was in x-ray, the patient's wife was sent to admitting to complete admission forms, sign permits, and prepare for admission of the patient and immediate surgery, pending results of x-rays and lab tests.

The scenario in Hospital Y (mission statement 2), however, would have proceeded as follows:

The physician was called. While waiting for the physician, the nurse called the admitting officer. The admitting officer interviewed the wife of the patient to determine insurance coverage and method of payment. Discovering that the patient had limited insurance coverage, the family was asked to fill out a financial statement. Based on this statement, the admitting officer determined that the patient should be transferred to the city hospital following emergency treatment and stabilization.

In the first scenario, the nurse's primary interaction was with the physician and family—the nurse's efforts were geared toward getting the patient admitted in an efficient and expeditious manner. My guess would be that the process was smooth, pleasant (for the family), and speedy.

In the second scenario, the nurse needed to add the admitting officer to her collaborative efforts. My guess is that in this situation the interface with the family was not smooth and pleasant, and certainly was not speedy.

So what is the point of all of this? First, the mission statement is significant to even the most common day-to-day nursing and patient care activity. Second, nursing input is important in mission/philosophy development. Third, mission and policy have an impact on collaborative relationships. Nurses cannot avoid organizational changes related to financial viability and must be aware of the impact of such changes on direct patient care and collaborative efforts and thus costs.

BUILDING INTERNAL COLLABORATIVE RELATIONSHIPS

One of the roles of the nurse executive as part of the executive management team is to educate administrative colleagues about what nurses do that makes a difference to patient outcome and recovery—not just patient welfare and comfort. When the chief executive officer asks the administrative group, "How can we deliver the same quality of care for $500 per day instead of $600 per day," the nurse executive's discussion might include nursing's contribution to decreasing length of stay, prevention of infection, patient/family compliance, and discharge planning.

Collaboration with administrative colleagues is definitely enhanced when the discussion by the nurse executive centers on how the team can work together to make the supply system work, and why the system *needs* to work for good patient care. The approach of "do it, because I said so" is long past. "I need your help" is better than "you've got a problem." It is important to keep in mind, however, that some members of the administrative team who have limited experience in health care institutions believe that as long as the physician orders it or the administrator requests it, it should be done. The most time-honored basis for minimizing the impact of this attitude has always been and continues to be—what is best for the patient. What is best for the patient is all health care givers and administrators collaborating for the patient's benefit.

Another key strategy for nurse executives to keep in mind to build administrative colleagueship is the "we/our" strategy. The financial problems are not *their* problems or the financial officer's problems, they are *our* problems. If "we" (total management team) share responsibility for the problems and the problem-solving decisions, then "we" can also share in the positive solutions.

In regard to justification of staffing increases, for example, an approach that includes only enhancement of programs and improved quality is no longer acceptable. Cost and revenue comparisons as well as the effect on the total organization are needed to complete the justification for new programs or continuing current programs. In order for the nurse executive to provide that data, a partnership, a colleagueship, a collaborative effort within the executive management team is essential. When faced with budget deficits, the basic approach to a budget reduction challenge begins with the following:

> We are all in this together—nursing staff, physicians, middle managers, and the entire executive management group. "I need your help" is the better approach than "you've got a problem."

Nothing is sacred except the patient. All programs must be evaluated in relation to their contribution to patient care versus cost of the program versus reimbursement level. No turf can be protected. All staff abilities and capabilities must be matched with patient needs.

For example, a clinician in a typical work day spends two hours with one client/family. In that two-hour period he or she accomplishes the following: secures supplies for home care until the return visit, sets a convenient time for the two-week return, helps the family obtain transportation home as well as for the return visit, confirms the home visit schedule with the local visiting nurse agency, and communicates with the local hospital emergency room regarding potential needs of the client. The cost, including clinician time, telephone, supplies, etc., versus the reduced cost of an additional stay in the hospital and the potential cost of an emergency visit provides the basis for establishing the appropriate positive value.

In contrast, if this same clinician spends the same two hours with ten clients, it would appear that the cost spread over ten patients (instead of one) would enhance the value and reduce the cost per patient, thus reducing the unit cost. If the analysis includes only cost per patient without analyzing the outcome of the encounter, a very important variable is missing. In this example, the encounter included a phone call to each client to check on the reason for missing a scheduled followup visit. The outcome was inconclusive, resulting in only one return visit, and it could have been carried out just as successfully by a clerk.

What does all this mean? In the latter example, the two hours and costs associated with the ten calls was wasted. It means that you might have the best clinician money can buy in helping families deal with the health care system, but a family may not perceive they have a need for this assistance (or the health care system) and for that matter may not be willing to pay for it. It then behooves the institution and the clinician to focus their energies where there is a perceived need, where the contribution of the service to patient welfare and for recovery is measurable, and where the service is cost-recoverable or cost-justified.

From another perspective, there is not a committee in the organization whose decisions do not have an impact on nursing directly or indirectly. For that reason, it is important to have nursing input into all organization interdepartmental committees.

Does the decision by the medical records committee to alter the chart format affect nursing? Does the decision by the utilization review committee to speed up the discharge planning process for chronic patients affect nursing? Does the decision of the pharmacy and therapeutics committee to move to a generic drug substitution policy affect nursing? The answer to all of these questions is, of course, yes. The bridges that the nurse manager builds through interdepartmental collaboration ensures that these issues are addressed with nursing's input.

Since nursing service interfaces with a multitude of internal support services, it also behooves the nurse executive to build collaborative relationships between his or her managers and those persons managing the internal support services. There is no other department or service within the hospital setting that depends on more departments or services than nursing. Therefore, it is imperative that relationships with these departments are established and maintained in a diplomatic and tactful manner if the nurse executive and the nurse managers are to achieve their goals and objectives.

EXTERNAL COLLABORATIVE RELATIONSHIPS

Peer collaboration external to the organization is also extremely important to nursing's future success. The nurse executive, or any nurse manager, needs support and feedback from colleagues in similar positions in other institutions. This author has always used colleagues locally and nationally for testing innovations, changing traditions, and ordinary day-to-day problem solving.

In the competitive environment in which we find ourselves, colleagueship nationally is even more critical. As institutions in the same locale compete for the same patients, the ability or desirability of discussing new program marketing strategies locally, for example, is lessened, and in many instances disappears. The colleagueship from out-of-state, out-of-market catchment areas, therefore, has become critical for survival.

The American Society for Nursing Service Administrators* provides the perfect forum for nurse executives to develop collegial relationships that lead to collaborative efforts nationally. In fact, the September–October 1984 bimonthly newsletter of the society reported on collaborative efforts being carried out between the society and the National Commission on Nursing "to promote further collaborative activities reflective of multiorganizational cooperation."[2] The newsletter also reported on separate activities with the American Association of Colleges of Nursing (AACN) and the Department of Health and Human Services in furthering collaborative efforts to enhance practice, education, and research issues.[3]

Through organizational activities, the author selected a colleague for consultation regarding primary nursing. Through a collaborative effort with a local colleague, we were able to bring our mutual colleague to our area to consult with our staff and ourselves.

Local collaborative efforts, although diminishing in breadth for reasons previously described, are still important and serve another worthwhile purpose. Joint efforts can accomplish professional and nursing community goals. For example, a citywide concern for baccalaureate completion programs for R.N.s spurred the nursing executive group of St. Louis into action. Their verbal and political support helped bring a B.S.N. completion program to St. Louis through the University of Missouri system.

Other issues that can and should be addressed by colleagues on a local level are: licensure issues (i.e., licensure of other health workers) and practice issues (such as revision of nurse practice acts). Specifically, proposed changes in L.P.N. practice related to their role in intravenous therapy has provided great opportunities in the state of Missouri for education, service, association, and state board of nursing collaborative efforts.

Collaborative efforts with local colleagues have also helped this author recruit national speakers for Professional Nurse Week, develop policies and procedures for a new program without reinventing the wheel, evaluate a staff reduction program, and keep sane during stressful periods. The latter cannot be emphasized too greatly. During internal crises, there is nothing more satisfying than to share the process of problem resolution with a colleague who has been there before. The necessity to test strategy, and gain confidence in the process, has become evident to this author. No

---

*The membership of ASNSA at its 1984 annual meeting in Chicago voted to rename the organization the American Organization of Nurse Executives.

problem is so large or so unique or so confidential that it cannot be shared with a trusted colleague. Common sense and the extent to which relationships have been nurtured help the nurse executive select the right colleague for the consultation needed.

In summary, the collaborative process (both internal and external to the organization) is vital as it relates to the achievement of success on the part of the nurse executive and nursing management to effect positive patient outcome and cost controls.

NOTES

1. Arthur X. Deegan and Thomas R. O'Donovan, *Management by Objectives,* 2nd ed. (Rockville, Md.: Aspen Systems Corp. 1982), p. 89.

2. American Society for Nursing Service Administrators, *Nursing Service Administration,* September-October 1984, p. 1.

3. American Society for Nursing Service Administrators, *Nursing Service Administration,* September-October 1984, p. 2.

Chapter 2

Collaborative Practice Models and Structures

Linda S. Cape, R.N., M.S.N.

INTRODUCTION

Throughout the past decade, the health care system at large has been subject to many changes and pressures. The health care consumer is demanding improved quality of care for all individuals at reduced costs. Physicians continue to feel overburdened with large case loads, rapidly changing technology, and malpractice concerns. Many physicians desire to meet their patients' needs and yet struggle with personal time constraints and with the necessity of relinquishing some patient care duties. Professional nurses are developing and expanding their roles in striving to provide improved and comprehensive care to patients and families. Yet they too struggle with these roles and ask questions as to whether the roles are the domain of nursing practice or medical practice. Other health care professionals also experience the pressures when attempting to determine and justify their individual roles in the various health care settings. The communities and agencies in which professionals provide care pose additional questions and concerns as to how the consumer can be served most efficiently and comprehensively at a reasonable cost.

All of these factors lead one to believe that there must be a better system for delivering quality health care in which the needs of the consumer are met, the skills of the health care professionals are utilized in an effective and efficient manner, health care costs are ultimately reduced, and satisfaction on the part of consumers, health care professionals, and institutions is maintained at a high level. That system can exist through the use of a collaborative practice model, which will be discussed in this chapter, along with ways that it can be adapted in various health care settings.

COLLABORATIVE PRACTICE MODEL

The collaborative practice model was first suggested in the early 1970s as a result of recommendations from the National Joint Practice Commission, which was established in 1971.[1] This commission was charged with examining the "roles and functions of physicians and nurses in providing high quality health care to the American people."[2] The commission focused its research on the relationships of physicians and nurses in hospitals and how these relationships enhanced or hindered the care of the patient and family. The collaborative practice model was developed and designed from these investigations and was successfully piloted in four different health care facilities. As a side note, in all of these facilities the model has been expanded to include other units within the hospital. These findings strongly support the many benefits afforded to patients, nurses, physicians, and the health care institution when collaborative practice is established.

Benefits

Some of the benefits of collaborative practice identified were: (1) patients reported increased satisfaction with the care they received; (2) nurses reported increased job satisfaction as they developed collegial relationships with physicians and as resultant patient care was provided in a more coordinated fashion; (3) physicians felt that patient satisfaction had improved and patients were better and more responsibly cared for; and (4) hospital administrators identified a vast improvement in the quality of patient care, an increase in patients' and professional staff's satisfaction, lowered indirect personnel costs, and ultimately lowered liability.[3] Thus it seems imperative that professionals within the health care system consider the concept of a collaborative practice model and adapt it to their individual setting.

What then is collaborative practice? Most simply defined, it is the joint determination of relationships among members of the health team whose sole purpose is to integrate their care practices into a comprehensive approach to meet the needs of patient and family. The definition seems simple enough, but to many of us in the health care community it may not be so simple to attain. Why not, we ask, when there are so many benefits?

Obstacles

There are several obstacles that must be addressed and confronted before collaborative practice can be implemented in any health care setting.

First one must determine if the health care environment is receptive to change. Each of us must examine our individual settings to determine answers to the following questions:

- Are nurses, physicians, and consumers satisfied with the level of care?
- Is there participation in decision-making issues by the team members?
- Is there a willingness for individuals to assume more responsibility?
- Are there concerns about job responsibilities?
- Are individuals satisfied with patient outcomes?
- Is there ongoing communication among health professionals?
- Do consumers receive consistent information regarding their health care needs?
- Is specific expertise utilized to the fullest potential?

For the health care institution, issues such as cost effectiveness, satisfaction of health care workers, and quality of care are generally of major concern. If these issues are currently being considered, discussed, and challenged in the health care environment, then most definitely these are seeds for change. Incorporating the concepts of change theory, foundations to support a model for collaborative practice can be laid.

A second obstacle, which is not generally addressed, is the direct relationship the development of a collaborative model has to the women's movement. Traditionally, nursing has been predominantly a female profession with the inherent so-called "feminine traits of being caring, tender, compassionate, having the presumed intuitive ability to relate to people, to be supportive of their needs and wants and thus be especially able to nurture others. Thus, women (nurses) should display specific behaviors because of these traits, i.e., being submissive, passive, subjective and emotional."[4]

On the other hand, physicians have predominantly been male with the so-called "masculine traits of being decisive, able to take initiative, being objective, persistent, aggressive, rational, brave and dominant."[5] Fortunately, although it is a slow evolution, females and males are increasing their numbers in the medical and nursing professions, respectively. However, because the evolution is slow, many of the archaic attitudes prevail, and there is conflict as nurses and physicians step out of their stereotyped roles.

Nurses are attempting to expand their roles through technical skill development, education, and research. The profession at large is coming into its own and nurses' struggle to be recognized as valuable and active participants in providing health care has been successful. With their advancing knowledge base, nurses are becoming more assertive in their communication and involvement with other health team members in an attempt to provide improved care. Some members of the nursing profession may see this evolution as a directional change toward becoming a miniphysician.

These nurses are very threatened by these changes as they require the nurse to be more responsible and more accountable for nursing actions and decisions. On the other hand, most nurses view these changes as an extremely positive movement toward the nursing profession being a valuable and recognizable contributor to the health care team.

Physicians also have differing viewpoints on the expanding nursing role. Some continue to view nurses as handmaidens who do not have the knowledge to participate in decision making regarding patient and family issues and are threatened by the nurse assuming what are characterized as "male traits." For example, the woman shouldn't be assertive or question physician directions: nurses are there to care and nurture the patient and not to cure. There are nurses as well who become very threatened when physicians show tenderness, caring, or emotion and don't respect that physician as they might another who is controlling, decisive, and so on. These traditional female-male roles continue to have some influence over how nurses and physicians relate in the health care environment. For the physician and nurse who continue to believe in these philosophies and are threatened by change, collaborative practice is more difficult to obtain. An important note, however, is that it is not impossible.

Fortunately, there are many physicians who are wholly supportive of developing collaborative relationships. These physicians are receptive to working with nurses and other team members to provide comprehensive care to the patient and family. They are not threatened by nurses' expanding roles and expertise, but in fact welcome the partnership and the sharing of responsibility and accountability. Nurses too are challenged to increase their knowledge and skill when they perceive that they are colleagues with the physicians and have important contributions to make in planning and delivering patient care and in facilitating patient recovery.

Prior to establishing a collaborative practice, physicians, nurses, and agency administrators must be aware that these obstacles are present but not insurmountable in the movement to implement a collaborative practice model.

ESTABLISHING COLLABORATIVE PRACTICE IN A HEALTH CARE FACILITY

The National Joint Practice Commission outlined five major steps that must be undertaken by physicians and nurses to establish collaborative practice in a health care setting.[6] These endeavors must have support from the administration: collaboration cannot be complete without this backing. Even though this model specifically focuses on the nurses and physicians collaborating in the hospital environment, it can be adapted easily to other health care settings and other health care professionals. Examples of these will be explored in greater depth in subsequent chapters.

The five elements that need to be addressed when establishing collaborative practice are: (1) establishing a joint practice committee; (2) implementing primary nursing as the nursing care delivery system; (3) encouraging nurses' individual clinical decision making; (4) integrating the patient record; and (5) conducting joint patient care record reviews. A discussion of each of these elements follows.

1. A joint practice committee is formed at the unit level, where there is equal representation of practicing nurses and physicians. Each member has equal weight in decision making regarding the policies regulating the nursing and medical practice on that unit. The committee is supported by the administration and continuously monitors nurse-physician relationships and recommends appropriate actions that foster and support collaborative practice.
2. Primary nursing is established as the mode for delivery of patient care. This is defined as the performance of clinical nursing functions performed by a professional nurse to a select group of patients and families with minimal delegation of nursing care functions to others. The primary nurse has a more thorough understanding of the patient's individualized needs and can enter more effectively into a collegial relationship with the physician(s) who provides the medical care to the patient.
3. Encouraging individualized decision making by nurses is vital for the collegial practice between nurses and physicians. If nurses are to utilize their professional skills to the fullest, they must be encouraged to make clinical nursing decisions based on the institution's scope of nursing practice as well as the nursing practice legislation in each state. Nurses are also encouraged to utilize medical and nursing consultants to enhance their decision making.
4. An integrated patient record is the fourth element necessary to establish a collaborative practice. An integrated record contributes to collaborative practice because it incorporates the observations, judgments, and actions of both the physician and the nurse and provides a formal means of communication. The nurse can easily identify the medical care plan and develop the nursing plan to enhance it. On the other hand, through the nurse's entries, the physician is aware of the nursing plan and how it contributes to facilitate patient recovery. Initially, nurses who are unfamiliar with charting in an integrated

record may feel inadequate communicating to physicians and other team members in this manner. They may lack confidence in their knowledge base and may feel that their nursing assessments and plans are not as important as the medical plans in affecting patient outcome. It is essential to support nurses by providing educational programs to help them build confidence in themselves and their profession and to develop skills in communication.

5. A joint review of the patient care record is the fifth element required for the establishment of collaborative practice. This consists of nurses and physicians reviewing together the patient care that they have provided. It is the critical step in determining if quality care was given. Through this mechanism, valuable feedback is given to nurses, physicians, and ultimately the administration regarding patient outcome, the quality of care being delivered, ways it can be maintained or improved, and cost factors reflected in decreased length of stay.

A comparison of the collaborative model with the traditional model is useful. The traditional model is reflected in Figure 2–1. The authority tends to flow in a downward direction with little exchange of ideas. Care is fragmented as different caregivers attempt to provide what they individually judge as being appropriate for the patient. The comprehensiveness and quality of care is in question as there is minimal communication between team members and the patient, with minimal evaluation of the care being provided. The end result is seen in few controls on costs or malpractice as care is disjointed.

Figure 2–1 Traditional Model

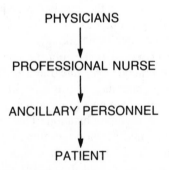

PHYSICIANS

PROFESSIONAL NURSE

ANCILLARY PERSONNEL

PATIENT

Source: Reprinted from *The American Journal of Medicine,* Vol. 74, p. 10, with permission of Technical Publishing Company, © 1983.

An example of the traditional model is as follows:

Mr. and Mrs. Smith had a premature infant who was admitted to the intensive care unit. The physician assessed the infant and family situation, spoke with the parents regarding the baby's problems, and developed a plan of care for the infant. The nurse and other health professionals met the parents, assessed the infant, and developed their individual plans of care. The health care professionals did not communicate with each other regarding their assessments of the family and infant and did not collaborate on the care plan.

As the hospitalization progressed, the infant developed complications related to the prematurity. His care was disjointed and fragmented because the nurse and physician did not collaborate on the therapy modes. The parents received inconsistent explanations and information about their infant from many health team members, and this heightened their anxiety. This anxiety led to increased hostility from the parents toward the staff and further frustrations for the staff members. The parents became so distrustful of the staff and fearful that their infant was not receiving quality care that they had the infant transferred to another facility. After the transfer of the infant, the parents initiated litigation proceedings against the physician and the admitting institution.

Thus, by functioning within the framework of the traditional model, the care was fragmented and communication was minimal, resulting in a malpractice suit.

The collaborative practice model represents a much different concept, as illustrated in Figure 2-2. The authority is not dictatorial: it includes a cooperative venture between the health care consumer and the other members of the team. There is much discussion and communication among the health team members to provide care in an integrated and comprehensive manner, thus ensuring a higher quality of care because of shared decision

Figure 2-2 Collaborative Practice Model

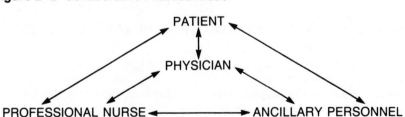

Source: Reprinted from *The American Journal of Medicine,* Vol. 74, p. 10, with permission of Technical Publishing Company, © 1983.

making. Evaluation of care is ongoing and incorporates feedback from all participants so that care can be adapted, and ultimately the needs of the patient can be met more efficiently and effectively. The end result with this model is that all team members share in controlling costs and malpractice litigation with the ultimate gain being improved patient outcome.

Taking the previous example of Mr. and Mrs. Smith, let us apply the collaborative practice model and observe how the situation would have been altered.

Mr. and Mrs. Smith had a premature infant who was admitted to the intensive care unit. The physician initially assessed the infant/family situation. The nurse and other team members then met to discuss their assessments and collaborate in developing a plan of care for both the infant and family. Thus, from the time of admission of the infant, the plan provided a comprehensive approach to care: consistent information was give to the parents; all team members were kept informed; and the care provided was of a higher quality as the expertise of various professionals was incorporated into the delivery of care.

As the hospitalization progressed, the infant developed complications related to his prematurity. The team of professionals continued to assess, collaborate, and evaluate the care. The parents were involved in the care of the infant, and team conferences were held with them to keep them informed of their infant's progress. The parents' anxiety was still present, but not to the degree noted in the first example. Throughout the hospitalization, the parents were given consistent information, participated in care, and received support from all team members, which helped to allay some of their fears. The infant was discharged to his parents at three months of age weighing 5 1/2 pounds.

The parents expressed much satisfaction with the care and support they had received for themselves as well as their infant. The staff also derived satisfaction in knowing that they had provided a comprehensive approach to meet the needs of the infant and family, which resulted in a positive outcome for the infant.

APPLYING THE MODEL TO OTHER PRACTICE AREAS

The collaborative practice model is a modern, practical approach to delivering health care. It has been developed with the primary area of implementation at the hospital facility and the development of relationships primarily between nurses and physicians. This model has a much broader applicability, not only to other disciplines within the health care system, but also to other health care environments.

The collaborative model also can be applied when considering how nursing works to interface within the institution. Figure 2–3 visually represents this collaborative relationship. The goals for the institution are jointly decided by representatives from both clinical nursing and nursing administration. Together these groups of individuals decide how to reach the goals and the timeframe in which they are to be accomplished. Thus, the first two criteria of the collaborative practice model have been attained: the two groups share responsibility for deciding the goals and have developed the manner in which they will be accomplished—the integrated approach. The approach is comprehensive because individuals from both groups bring their expertise in considering different options and solving problems. Specifically, at Children's Hospital in St. Louis, this collaboration begins at the unit level with staff nurses and the unit managers deciding on unit goals. From this level, it transcends to the administrative board level. Chapter 1 discusses this in further detail.

Nursing collaborating with nursing can utilize this model whether it is at the clinical practice level, at the nursing education level, or at the nursing research level. At the clinical practice level, the staff nurse may collaborate with other staff nurses to develop the plan of care, provide the care in an integrated and comprehensive manner, and evaluate the outcome of the care. This format of care is primary nursing, where the primary nurse and associate care nurses take responsibility for a patient and family to provide quality nursing care (see Figure 2–4). In another form of clinical practice the format may incorporate a nursing consultant or clinical nurse specialist who collaborates with the staff nurses to develop the care plan.

Nurses collaborating with nurse educators and researchers is another way in which the collaborative model can be adapted. The ultimate goal is to enhance and improve the quality of care delivered to the patient. Thus, with education it may mean the clinical nurse specialist working with nurse educators to develop a curriculum that is more appropriate to health care needs and to day-to-day clinical practice situations. The educator and specialist share responsibility in developing and teaching a curriculum that is of a higher quality and more comprehensive as it includes both dimensions of

---

Figure 2–3 Nursing-Institution Collaborative Relationship

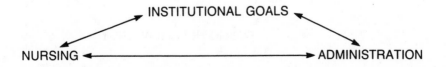

Figure 2–4 Primary Nursing Model

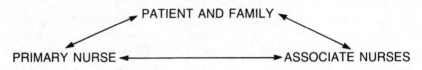

practice. The outcome is a nurse who is better prepared to practice in society and a nursing profession that can assure the public of higher quality professional nurses. (See Chapter 6 for further discussion.)

The nurse researchers collaborating with nurses in clinical practice use the model as well. It is only through communication between these two groups that nursing care problems and issues can be approached and solved systematically. Through collaboration, the problems are jointly identified and discussed, a comprehensive plan of investigation is developed, and the outcome affects the quality of patient care.

Using the collaborative model to work with other team members, whether they are within the hospital setting or another setting, has been addressed with the initial discussion of the model. Further exploration of this concept will be discussed in Chapter 8. Let it suffice to say that through collaboration the team members have shared participation and responsibility. The leader of the team will change as dictated by the needs of the patient; thus it is not a static system, but a fluid one.

How can the collaborative practice model be adapted to the nurse in the community? Depending on the specific system, the individuals vary, but the model remains constant. For example, consider the public health nurse. As noted in Figure 2–5, there is communication among all members where patient needs are assessed and a specific plan of care is developed. With

Figure 2–5 Public Health Nurse Model

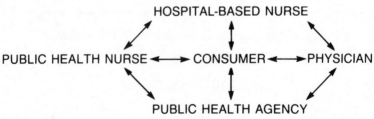

participation of all members, the approach is integrated and care is provided in an efficient and effective manner. Throughout the management of care, there are periodic evaluations and redirection of care based on consumer needs. Without the use of collaboration in this setting, there is inevitable overlap of services, with a disjointed approach resulting in poorer quality of care and increase in costs. The key is mutual agreement on the plan of care and thus a holistic approach to the consumer.

For nurses who are providing care with the physician in private practice, the collaborative practice model is essential. In this situation, the nurse and physician must agree on nursing and medical areas of practice, develop basic trust and mutual respect for each other, and be willing to share responsibility for the quality of care being delivered. Many professionals identify this system of patient care as "joint practice." I do not differentiate this from the model of collaborative practice: the elements are identical. The practice area is predominantly in the community versus the hospital environment.

Along this continuum, nurses who choose to practice independently within the community (i.e., nurse midwives, nurse practitioners) are not wholly independent because they, too, utilize the collaborative practice model by working with a consulting physician. These nurses manage and provide the primary care for their clientele; however, they refer to their consulting physician when warranted by specific patient situations. On the other hand, the physician also refers patients to the nurses when they can be managed within the nurses' realm of expertise. Without collaboration between the physicians and nurses, independent practice is difficult to develop and maintain.

A third example of collaboration in the community is the nurse working with other agencies or institutions in the community (see Figure 2-6). It may be demonstrated in the following example: the nurse from the hospital collaborates with the school system to facilitate the re-entry into the educational system of a child who has a chronic illness.

Again, the concept of collaboration is necessary to ensure that the child is provided with ongoing education and at the same time that his or her

Figure 2-6 Nurse/Community Collaboration

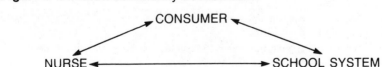

medical needs are being met. Without collaboration, the educators are uncomfortable having a child with special needs in their classrooms, the child's education is compromised, and his feelings of self-worth and ultimately his medical condition deteriorate.

SUMMARY

The collaborative practice model can be adapted to all areas of practices. The professionals, institutions, and systems involved vary, but the primary focus—providing quality care to the consumer—remains constant. With this model, the care is provided in a comprehensive manner where quality is maintained, costs are contained, and professionals derive satisfaction as their individual skills and expertise are appropriately used. To ensure that this model is the basis of our health care delivery system, we as nurse professionals must strive to educate our future physicians, nurses, and other health professionals in its concept. It is a vital component for the health care system of the future.

NOTES

1. The National Joint Practice Commission, *Guidelines for Establishing Joint or Collaborative Practice in Hospitals* (Chicago, Ill.: Neely Printing Co, Inc., 1981), pp. 1–31.

2. Ibid., p. 1.

3. Ibid., pp. 4–6.

4. Wilma S. Hiede, "Nursing and Women's Liberation: A Parallel," *American Journal of Nursing*, May 1973, p. 824.

5. Ibid.

6. The National Joint Practice Commission, *Guidelines for Establishing Joint or Collaborative Practice in Hospitals* (Chicago, Ill.: Neely Printing Co., Inc., 1981), p. 4.

SUGGESTED READINGS

Adelson, Bernard, and Werner, June. "Fostering Collaborative Relationships." *The Hospital Medical Staff*, March 1981, pp. 5–10.

American Nurses' Association. *Nursing: A Social Policy Statement*. Kansas City, Mo.: American Nurses' Association, 1980.

Ardine, Carolyn R., and Pridham, Karen F. "Model for Collaboration." *Nursing Outlook* 21 (1973): 655–657.

Batt, William L., Jr., and Weinberg, Edgar. "Labor Management Cooperation Today." *Harvard Business Review* 56 (1978): 96–104.

Bennis, Warren G.; Benne, Kenneth S.; and Chin, Robert. *The Planning of Change*. New York: Holt, Rinehart and Winston, Inc., 1969.

Blackwood, Sarah, and Ryker, David. "Establishing the Collaborative Practice Committee." *The Hospital Medical Staff* 10 (March 1981): 11–16.

Bruton, Dana L. "Following the NJPC Guidelines," in *Persuading Physicians*. Edited by Robert Rubright. Rockville, Md.: Aspen Systems Corp., 1984, pp. 109–112.

Burchell, R. Clay; Thomas, Debra A.; and Smith, Howard L. "Some Considerations for Implementing Collaborative Practice." *The American Journal of Medicine* 74 (1983): 9–13.

Burke, Lora E. "The Clinical Nurse Specialist in Collaborative Practice." *Momentum: American Nurses' Association Council of Clinical Nurse Specialists* 1 (1983): 3–5.

Cape, Linda S. "The Clinical Nurse Specialist," in *Coping with Caring for Sick Newborns*. Edited by R.E. Marshall, C. Kasman, and L.S. Cape. Philadelphia: W.B. Saunders Co., 1982, pp. 145–161.

DeRose, Joseph. "Implementing the Basic Elements of Collaborative Practice." *The Hospital Medical Staff*, March 1981, pp. 19–25.

Devereux, Pamela McNutt. "Essential Elements of Nurse-Physician Collaboration," *The Journal of Nursing Administration*, May 1981, pp. 19–23.

Devereux, Pamela McNutt. "Nurse/Physician Collaboration: Nursing Practice Considerations." *The Journal of Nursing Administration*, September 1981, pp. 37–39.

England, Doris. "Creating a Climate for Solutions: A Nursing Administrator's Perspective," in *Coping with Caring for Sick Newborns*. Edited by R.E. Marshall, C. Kasman, and L.S. Cape. Philadelphia: W.B. Saunders Co., 1982.

Grissum, M., and Spengler, C. *Womanpower and Health Care*. Boston: Little, Brown and Co., 1976.

Heide, Wilma S. "Nursing and Women's Liberation: A Parallel." *American Journal of Nursing* 73 (1973): 824–827.

Lewis, Mary Ann. "Climate for Collaboration," in *Persuading Physicians*. Edited by Robert Rubright. Rockville, Md.: Aspen Systems Corp., 1984, pp. 101–107.

Mamana, John P. "New Concept Has Promise." *The Hospital Medical Staff*, March 1981, pp. 2–4.

Mauksch, Ingeborg G. "Nurse-Physician Collaboration: A Changing Relationship." *The Journal of Nursing Administration*, June 1981, p. 35–38

Mauksch, Ingeborg G. "Nurse-Physician Collaboration: A Changing Relationship," in *Nursing in Transition*. Edited by T. Audean Duesphol. Rockville, Md.: Aspen Systems Corp., 1983, pp. 233–238.

Philips, John R. "Health Care Provider Relationships: A Matter of Reciprocity." *Nursing Outlook*, November 1979, pp. 738–741.

Reed, John M.; Neblett, Peter; and Neblett, Randy. "Using An Integrated Physician-Nurse Medical Record." *The Hospital Medical Staff*, March 1981, pp. 26–30.

Shumaker, Denese, and Gost, Virginia. "Toward Collaboration: One Small Step." *Nursing and Health Care*, November 1980, pp. 183–185.

Steel, John E. "Putting Joint Practice Into Practice." *American Journal of Nursing*, May 1981, pp. 964–969.

The National Joint Practice Commission. *Guidelines for Establishing Joint or Collaborative Practice in Hospitals*. Chicago, Ill.: Neely Printing Co., Inc., 1981.

Vaughan, Ruth A. "Collaborative Practice." *Nursing Management* 13 (1982): 33–35.

Winker, Cynthia Kelsey, and Lee, Nancy C. "Developing a Joint Practice Team." *Dimensions of Critical Care Nursing* 1 (1982): 360–363.

Wise, Harold; Rubin, Irwin; and Beckard, Richard. "Making Health Teams Work." *American Journal of Diseases of Children* 127 (1974): 537–542.

Part II

Chapter 3

Environment for Collaborative Practice/Professionalism

Amy Hemme Kennedy, R.N., M.S.N.

INTRODUCTION

This chapter discusses the necessary components that make up a collaborative environment. Five areas are discussed: the contemporary women's movement, executive modeling, decentralized organizational structure, expanded roles in nursing, and primary nursing. When any one of these five components is missing in an organization, collaborative relationships are discouraged, and personnel become frustrated.

The concepts of leadership, responsibility, accountability, assertiveness, risk-taking, and autonomous interventions are discussed throughout as they apply to collaborative practice in each section of the chapter.

WOMEN'S EMERGING ROLE: BACKDROP FOR COLLABORATION

The socialization of women to be only wives and mothers has dramatically changed in the last 20 years. Currently women can enter any field they choose and excel in it. Sex differentiation of roles is less and less a factor. Equal education and equal opportunity are more the norm.

In the mid-1980s, when one looks at the environment for collaboration, one need pause only a moment to realize that our sociocultural environment is an asset. The women's movement, which emerged as an organized front in the mid-1960s, has helped to set this stage. Today women are viewed as individuals with valid ideas, knowledge, and skill.

The 1970s saw feminism as rhetoric give way to practical demands by women entering the work force in record numbers. This changed role of women has affected both men and women in the home and on the job.

Since 1950, the number of women working outside the home has nearly tripled. Around 15 percent of families are headed by women, and in nearly 6 million homes wives earn more than their husbands.[1]

Women have made significant advances in almost every field. Their numbers are increasing rapidly as they become doctors, lawyers, administrators, politicians, professors, stockbrokers, architects, engineers, pilots, and bankers. Role models are all around us: Geraldine Ferraro, vice presidential candidate; Supreme Court Justice Sandra Day O'Connor; and Transportation Secretary Elizabeth Dole.

Women are also going to the voting booth and the court house to bring about economic and social reform in employment, insurance and pension plans, divorce settlements, and child care arrangements. They are running for office at national, state, and local levels and winning.

The period of establishing a family overlaps with the period of establishing a career, and one must learn to juggle competing demands. As women try to do both, marriage roles have changed. Women are getting married later and having fewer children, and adequate child care becomes a critical issue. Career women need to know they can depend on their husbands and on quality child care.

Even with all the stress, there are indicators that many women are successfully combining work and family. The fear of working women being at greater risk for heart attacks, mid-life breakdowns, and shortened life-spans have not been borne out. Women still have only half the chance of developing heart disease that men have. Studies also show that women's mental health has improved. The incidence of depression in women between the ages of 35–55 has declined dramatically in the last ten years. The health-promoting aspects of work seem to offset the stress.

The advent of the contraceptive pill has enabled women to plan their families with more ease. Since 1960 the birth rate has been halved. The number of women in their thirties having their first baby has tripled since 1970.[2]

The changes in women's roles are also showing up in books, films, and on television. Women are appearing as wage earners, leaders, and heads of households instead of housewives or men chasers.[3]

The women's movement has been a catalyst in our society to bring about change, and this change is a facilitator of collaboration. One of the specific ways collaboration is enhanced in the health care field is the emphasis on assertiveness. Women generally, and nurses specifically, have learned better ways to speak up and communicate their point of view. Through workshops, conferences, and support groups, women have grown to express what they think in an unemotional nonaggressive way that is listened to and respected. This skill is basic to collaboration.

Networking is another skill learned by women as a necessity as they enter the business world. *Webster's New World Dictionary* defines networking as "a system of interconnected or cooperating individuals." Women who previously had been content to get ahead on their own began to appreciate the advantages of making and using contacts. They "called in favors" from other women they met socially in the community or at work. In turn, these women called on them. Soon they realized that, over time, they had established a large number of individual contacts to whom they could turn for information, advice, support, or access to others. Networking itself is a collaborative effort and leads to further collaboration as information gleaned from one level of contact feeds into another.[4]

However, many women find that while they are intellectually capable, they are often emotionally unprepared for the situations they encounter. The competitiveness, the power politics, and the need for constant assertion of one's identity all present special problems to individuals who have traditionally been in the background. Added to this are the complications that develop if a professional woman marries and has children. Some seek help because of symptoms brought on by stress, such as severe anxiety, apprehension, and panic; some are depressed and some have psychosomatic symptoms.

Women are now working with goals different from those they had formerly. They are choosing to pursue a career as part of their sense of identity. This is the important distinction. What has been called "identity work" was formerly restricted almost exclusively to men. A woman's identity was traditionally defined by marriage and family, as wife and mother. A man's identity was primarily defined by his work, with marriage and family giving him the necessary nurturance and support.

Women who enter professions now do not plan to drop out for marriage and family. They are becoming deeply involved in their work and look forward to further career development plus family. Now that women are seeking self-actualization through work, they are confronted with specific conflicts that cause anxiety and that must be resolved.

One great source of conflict occurs because many women are not prepared for the ordinary aggressive and competitive atmosphere they find in many areas of their career.

A second source of anxiety and conflict is the widespread fears that many women have concerning competence. As they become more competent, they often panic because they experience this as a loss of femininity.

A third area of conflict occurs in their relationships with men—boyfriends or husbands—and in their function as mothers. As women become less compliant and submissive, they meet various reactions from the men close to them, often causing friction that they are unable to handle effectively. As they become more identified with their work, they find that they are less willing and less able to subordinate their professional activities to husband and children without considerable inner turmoil.[5]

Coping with these conflicts is a challenge, and individual professional women find individual ways to bring their family, work, and friends into balance. Friendship and support from other professional women is very helpful, as well as organized support groups that help with values clarification and mutual problem solving. The recent emphasis on good nutrition and exercise for stress reduction has been very useful to many professional women as well.

As the next generation is being socialized into more equal educational experiences and equal opportunities throughout our culture, some of this anxiety will disappear. However, the juggling act between home, family, and career will continue.

EXECUTIVE MODELING: SETTING THE STAGE FOR COLLABORATION WITHIN AN ORGANIZATION

To establish an environment for collaboration, it is important to have leadership in a department of nursing that is on a parity with other leadership within the hospital organization. Executive modeling to the entire nursing staff is the key in setting a tone for collaboration with other health care professionals. The leadership that the executive models is very specific: it defines the roles of self and others in relationship to goal achievement, structures and interprets the situation to the group in an ongoing way, and shows respect and consideration for the ideas of other group members and other people in the department and throughout the organization.[6]

One of the recent studies done by the American Academy of Nursing, *Magnet Hospitals: Attraction and Retention of Professional Nurses,* speaks to this issue.[7] This study looks at hospitals across the country that succeed in attracting and retaining professional nurses. The study's aim was to describe the factors associated with this success. Both the nurse executive and a staff nurse at each participating hospital were interviewed.

The administrative factors that appear to allow participating hospitals to attract and retain nurses were: management style, quality of leadership, organizational structure, staffing, and personnel policies. Specific characteristics were:

1. Magnet hospitals practice participative management, and communication flows in both directions.

2. There is an unbroken chain of able and qualified leaders at each organization level, and nursing leaders are regarded as risk-takers in achieving their goals.
3. Meaningful philosophy of patient care permeates day-to-day operations.
4. Nursing staff believes they are supported by nursing administration, and the latter believes the same about hospital administration.
5. Most magnet hospitals are decentralized, providing a sense of control at the nursing unit level.
6. There is heavy nurse involvement in the hospital committee structure.
7. Staffing is adequate in quantity and quality.
8. Salaries and benefits are competitive with other hospitals in the community.
9. Managers try hard to accommodate the personal lives of staff when devising work schedules.
10. There are promotional systems that recognize clinical expertise.

As one looks at these ten areas one sees that there is a high regard for the profession of nursing, the practice of nursing, and the individual nurse. This kind of administrative structure allows the nurse to begin practice, grow in the practice, and become expert in that practice. With this kind of environment, self-confidence and self-esteem as an individual and as a professional are promoted, which is the groundwork for collaborative practice on a health care team. If persons feel confident in their professional roles and with their peer professionals, they can take that confidence into the interdisciplinary arena and collaborate effectively on the health care team. When elements of the above-mentioned administrative structure are absent, i.e., participative management structure or support from the nurse executive, the practicing nurse becomes frustrated, and diminished self-esteem and self-respect as a professional acts as a deterrent to collaborative practice.

The nurse executive who sets the tone for collaborative practice performs a number of interacting functions. Mintzberg, as discussed by Stevens, has identified ten major roles executives play:

1. Figurehead (functioning as symbolic formal head of the division filling ceremonial functions).
2. Leader (directing subordinates to goal achievement and motivating and working with staff).
3. Liaison (building a communication network, establishing contacts outside the vertical chain of command).

4. Monitor (scanning the environment for information pertinent to the job, keeping abreast of changes in the power structure or the organization direction).
5. Disseminator (sharing and distributing information with staff, determining what goes to whom, where, and why).
6. Spokesperson (speaking for the division, addressing key external and internal publics).
7. Entrepreneur (looking for improvement opportunities, taking the initiative in new projects and developments).
8. Disturbance Handler (mediating and resolving disputes and disruptions among work groups).
9. Resource Allocator (determining how the division's resources are to be distributed).
10. Negotiator (managing formalized and informal bargaining with both internal and external groups).[8]

To perform these interacting functions effectively, nurse executives need to be flexible, innovative, and caring, as well as have a great deal of self-awareness. To be aware of characteristics such as the degree of maturity they have (maturity is defined as a willingness and ability to do a task), nurse executives must be aware of their motivation and knowledge base regarding the task. Motivation is vital to effective leadership. Being a leader is a large task, and it involves not only the willingness and ability to accept responsibility for oneself, but also for actions of the group one is leading. Having a solid knowledge base in administrative nursing is also key for nurse executives. They need broad information in the health care field within the organization, within the community, and within the nation as a whole to be effective leaders.[9]

Being able to set goals is another area that the nurse executive needs to model for those in the department. Many things are necessary to achieve goals, like time, money, and persons, and within these limitations goals must be sound and realistic. Goals also need to be set in short-term and long-term timeframes. Most importantly, the nurse executive needs to be able to communicate these goals to the managers in the department and help them set short- and long-term goals to accomplish the larger goals. In the current environment of cost-containment, the nurse executive has an even greater challenge to help managers be fiscally responsible as they set short- and long-range goals.

Awareness of power is also critical for the leader who is setting the stage for collaboration. How it is used and how it is achieved is very important. Leaders must recognize that they have power. It may be achieved by virtue of the position or it may be achieved by trust relationships within the organization. The interactions of leader and members help to establish a group power base that can be directed toward goal achievement, which in the long run has much more power, much more effect, than just the traditional use of power.

Nurse executives also need to be aware of their personalities and how they are viewed by others. Leaders need to know the extent of their self-confidence, enthusiasm, flexibility, creativity, honesty, sincerity, tact, and friendliness, since this awareness will lead to a clearer understanding of how they affect others.

Knowledge of assets and liabilities in one's personal appearance is also important to be aware of how one's appearance influences a group. Communication skills are very critical for the leader, and the basic goal is to convey a clear straightforward message to the group and to be sensitive to the response the message elicits from the group. An awareness of both the leader's and the group's verbal and nonverbal communication behavior is very important.[10]

Nurse executives need to be aware of their physical and emotional limits. The stresses of executive modeling are very great, and therefore there must be an awareness of how stress is managed. It is important for the leader to be able to say "yes" and "no" and to do so in such a way that the persons presenting the ideas or the proposal will not be offended personally but will understand the broad range of information the nurse executive has and the reasons for the positive or negative answer.

Knowing each individual within the group helps the nurse executive to predict the goals, needs, abilities, and values as well as the strengths, limitations, and potential of the whole group. For the group to work together, each individual member must fuse into the group. The leader facilitates this fusion by having empathy for each individual member.

Communication among group members is essential for any productive work to occur. Therefore, the nurse executive must be aware of the communication patterns within the group, and the group leader becomes a facilitator. Group members' satisfaction increases as the frequency of consultation initiated by the leader increases; that is, group members like to be asked about their opinions and approaches to situations in which they are expected to participate. This kind of self-awareness is basic at the top level for collaboration throughout the whole organization. If nurse executives model these behaviors, most of the people in their group will learn these skills.

Assertiveness is another important attribute for the nurse executive. Assertiveness includes expressing one's feelings, needs, and ideas and standing up for one's rights while considering the rights of others. Assertive persons establish close interpersonal relationships, protect themselves from being used by others, make their own life decisions and choices, identify and meet many of their interpersonal needs, and express positive and negative feelings both verbally and nonverbally. Assertive persons generally feel good about themselves and others. Assertive behavior is a basic characteristic to be found in a nurse executive as well as a manager and is key to collaborative relationships at all levels of the organization and between nursing and other disciplines.[11]

Accountability is another attribute of the effective leader. Leaders are accountable to themselves, their group, their profession, and their superiors. Accountability is answering to someone for the positive or negative outcomes of one's actions. To be accountable to themselves, persons must be able to view objectively what they are doing with their work and their lives. Persons must feel satisfied with what they are doing to be effective leaders. Accountability includes negative as well as positive elements. Accountability to one's profession includes a willingness to judge one's professional peers and a conscientious development of the ability to judge. Accountability to one's superiors includes goal achievement and goal evaluation on an ongoing basis.[12]

Finally, effective leaders are always advocates for their group. An advocate supports and defends someone or something. Advocacy has been called that part of a person's nature known as selfish benevolence. In other words, an advocate assists a group to achieve and use power effectively to produce certain desired societal changes.

The executive modeling discussed above has to be emulated and modeled to the staff nurse level as well. In a study reported in *Nursing '78*, "Job Satisfaction—Or Should That Be Dissatisfaction?," questionnaires were sent to nurses all over the country in regard to immediate managers' feedback. The results reported that only about one-third of the nurses felt that they were receiving adequate constructive feedback from their nurse manager.[13] The refrain in the returned letters was unmistakable—nurses wanted more interaction with their managers about the quality of their work, both in terms of affirmation and in terms of correction. Some indicated that they actually left their jobs because they felt they were doing more and more and no one paid any attention to it. One nurse said, "When I handed in my resignation, the evaluation made me look like a super-nurse, and if I had had that kind of feedback earlier, I might have stayed."

Fortunately, patients show their appreciation. More than 70 percent of the nurses that responded to the questionnaire felt that the patients understood what the nurses were doing for them and expressed their appreciation. One of the reported themes from this study was that nursing administration does not get its information across very well. About 35 percent of the staff nurses thought communication between administration and the staff level was good, whereas 80 percent of nursing administration thought it was good or excellent. This disparity indicates some lack of understanding and communication on both parts.[14]

One of the ways to motivate people is to support them when they run into problems. The study from *Nursing '78* indicates that 51 percent of the respondents received support frequently or most of the time, 30 percent occasionally, and 19 percent seldom. Thirteen percent reported a great deal of faith in their hospital administration, 40 percent a fair amount, 24 percent little, and 23 percent very little. The respondents seem to appreciate the financial problems of running an institution, but the consensus was that management does not deal effectively with big problems and actually creates petty ones.[15] Obviously, these nurses are speaking out for collaboration, a greater share in decision making, and support from their superiors.

Thus the nurse executive needs to create a team approach throughout the whole department of nursing. The nurses need to feel that they are in the organization for the same reason—mainly to care for sick people and help them regain their health and manage their health problems in the best way possible. A team approach can only be accomplished when the channels of communication are open, and communication is from the bottom up as well as the top down. Open communication is based on genuine respect of the nurse executive by his or her staff and a mutual respect by the nurse executive of the people making up the team. This collegiality is described by Margretta Styles. (See also Chapter 5.)

> Collegiality, the sharing of responsibility and authority with our colleagues, is an attitude about our individual nurse-to-nurse relationships. It is based on ultimacy and leads to respect. The first recognizes that doing nursing work to the utmost is enhanced by an appropriate collaborative effort—recognizes that through genuine collaboration, individual endeavor is potentiated, not just pooled. Respect then follows with the acknowledgement and encouragement of the contribution that others made toward a mutual task. . . . Collegiality 1) de-emphasizes status differences in responsibility and authority—the test organizes the work; leadership and fellowship fluctuate; 2) focuses on the functional rather than dysfunctional aspect of individual performance, and accepts foibles; 3) promotes sharing of information and recognizes this as necessary for task accomplishment as well as individual growth— this ranges from personal reporting on one level to scholarly communication through professional journals on another; 4) takes seriously the opinions of others—hears dissent objectively; 5) takes seriously the work of others and builds on it; 6) values peer review and both offers and receives constructive criticism; 7) encourages

risk-taking in oneself and others by joint problem solving and mutual support; 8) stresses remediation rather than blame setting or blame avoidance.[16]

Clearly, collaboration from the executive level is necessary to support collaborative practice in nursing.

DECENTRALIZED ORGANIZATIONAL STRUCTURE

One of the essential components for collaborative practice is a decentralized organization, where patient care decisions are made at the unit level. This system demands strong leadership from first-line managers, as discussed previously. In most organizations, these people are called head nurses, clinical directors, or patient care managers. They need sound nursing knowledge as well as a good understanding of management theory. The responsibilities include planning for staffing and equipment, maintaining the environment on a unit, and working with all the departments that interface with the patients and staff on a unit. This is a large order, and traditionally the nurses doing this job have learned it from their predecessors or from observing other good managers rather than from a theoretical base. More recently nurses are taking management courses at the graduate level for nurse management positions, which provides a sounder theory base from which to practice.

The person in first-line management also has budgetary responsibilities. The patient care manager (or head nurse) is responsible for the budget for his or her particular unit, which requires negotiating with the nurse executive and the hospital administrator for the necessary staff positions, equipment, and disposable goods that are required to take care of patients on the unit. As stated previously, the current environment of cost-containment focuses much more activity and creativity on this area of management than ever before.

Along with the budgeting for the staff is the actual interviewing and hiring, orienting, supervising, evaluating, and terminating, if that is necessary. A nurse manager in a decentralized organization may have 30 to 130 nurses in his or her employ and is also responsible for providing resources for continuing education for these people after they are on the job. All of this requires expert communication skills, expert clinical knowledge, and expert managerial skills to run a smooth patient care unit in an effective, efficient way. Visible acceptance of responsibility for management decisions at the higher levels of the hierarchy conveys a message to the first-line manager that acknowledges the risk inherent in decision making. If superiors are risk-takers, the patient care manager will feel safer accepting such risk in running a unit. Responsibility needs to be clarified at all levels of the hierarchy.[17]

Authority is another important aspect of the first-line manager position. Authority has to include the power to act. Individuals at all levels who have been allocated and who have accepted responsibility must be authorized to handle the functions for which they are being held responsible, and they need to decide how to carry out those functions. Congruence between responsibility and authority is vitally important and must be thought out carefully. Lack of congruence between these elements results in lack of clearly understood decision making.

The nurse manager is also accountable for decisions within the broad scope of the health care field. Accountability in the nursing profession deals with the act of providing a nursing service to a designated individual or group of individuals. In order for an individual to be held accountable or responsible for nursing action, a safety or quality standard must exist as a criterion of measurement. The American Nurses' Association (ANA) established criteria of measurement in 1975 when the Congress for Nursing Practice formulated the Standards for Nursing Practice. Accountability is defined by Webster as "the quality or state of being accountable, liable and responsible," and another definition from Webster states that to be accountable means to be "answerable."[18] These definitions suggest that someone other than oneself judges the degree of fulfillment of specific obligations. In a decentralized nurse management environment, this accountability weighs heavily on the nurse manager, who is responsible for a geographic unit 24 hours a day and the people who staff that unit 24 hours a day. The nurse manager is also responsible for encouragement of professional growth and development in the individual nurse through inservice education at the unit level or within the hospital setting and at specific conferences or seminars that relate to the appropriate area of practice.

First-line management serves as a link between the nurse executive and nursing staff. Nurse managers act as an active conduit of messages throughout the nursing organization, carrying goals, policies, and purposes downward to staff and monitoring information up to the nurse executive. Furthermore, the first-line manager must serve as an authority and consultant concerning means by which staff nurses may meet executive-determined ends. In addition, first-line managers will evolve their own goals specific to their areas of managerial responsibility. This mutual goal-setting effort requires collaborative skill on the part of the first-line manager.

A second linking function comes into focus as first-line managers know a wider world than does the typical staff nurse. They have knowledge of the institution beyond that of the nursing unit. They also know what people in what departments may be useful in problem solving as well as appropriate community resources. One of their major teaching functions is to introduce the staff nurse to a greater expanse of resources than those of the unit. Modeling collaboration with this broader health care team is invaluable to the staff nurse's role development.

The primary domain for first-line management decisions lies with nursing systems and their nurse managers rather than with patients or staff. First-line managers should be systems analysts, seeing that supply lines, communication systems, and systems of care delivery function at peak performance. They facilitate getting the work done by providing the environment in which that is possible. The logistic questions in a complex institution are difficult and require more than incident-by-incident patchwork attention. First-line managers are ideally equipped to deal with systems problems; they have a good overview of the functioning of the total organization, or at least a good portion of it.

The other major responsibility of first-line managers is upward to the top nurse executive. First-line management is responsible for conveying the state of the department to the executive level. This assignment must be accurate for effective planning by top management. Just as first-line management is responsible for development of staff, so is executive management responsible for further development of those first-line managers who have potential for executive management. Often this potential is recognized and developed by allowing first-line management to participate in or observe executive management decision making and goal setting.

Another necessary ingredient for collaboration is an attitude within an organization that "anything's possible," and that change is welcome rather than resisted. Nursing leadership needs to demonstrate flexibility in innovative thinking and planning to accommodate the variety of needs of individual staff and of the whole patient care environment. There is much rigidity and bureaucracy in health care, and we need to foster innovative solutions. When we think of change we think of planned change and unplanned change. With planned change, the change agent, or the person desiring to bring about change, can be from within the organization or from without. The likelihood of success of planned change is greater when the change agent is known within the organization and respected professionally and personally.

As well as flexibility within the organization and adequately prepared change agents at appropriate levels to create change and to bring it about, an environment conducive to collaboration must also include an awareness of professional trends within the community and nation. The nurse executive, first-line management, and clinical management need to be exposed to literature and conference speakers who are trend setters for professional nursing and then bring information back into the organization as new ideas and new ways of doing things. Well-informed nursing staff aware of what is going on in other parts of the country and in other health institutions within the same city are in a much better position to collaborate with other professionals on the health care team in bringing about improved patient care.

Another important aspect of openness to change is the ability on the part of management to say that something does not work. Perhaps it's a good idea, but now is not the time; then stop it and go back to the previous method. This takes courage and confidence, but it is better to say, "now is not the right time," or recognize that something is not working rather than to let it continue and decrease morale and create problems within the organization.

When creating change within an organization, staffing should be evaluated to see if it is adequate to accomplish the work. This includes time available for the creative process of starting something new and bringing about change. Resource people who are prepared at advanced levels, who know change theory and other theoretical frameworks, also need to be available. Planning for change is a very important aspect of an organization's ongoing activity. Management By Objectives, or another management system, builds in a mechanism whereby problems are identified and problem-solving activities follow to direct the organization's energy. This kind of system also builds in target dates for accomplishment and for periodic evaluations. This occurs at the executive level, first-line management level, and staff level so that there is planned change activity going on at all times.

Although resistance to change is expected among large numbers of persons who did not participate in the planning of the proposed change, their importance goes beyond the role of resisters, because a necessary prerequisite of successful change involves the mobilization of the forces against it. Two principles of implementation outlined by Benuviste can be used by nursing leaders to foster implementation of the desired change by mobilizing and redirecting the forces within the opposing group. The first principle is that implementation is likely to occur only when the system of rewards and punishments operates in a manner that encourages implementation. The second principle is the multiplier effect, which refers to the reality that it is difficult to oppose a course of action that appears to be inevitable. If a plan is announced, but people continue to be rewarded for doing something else, the plan will probably not be implemented. This simple statement explains the need for the system of rewards and punishments to be altered in such a way as to foster implementation of the desired change.[19]

A decentralized organizational structure sets the stage for collaboration by allowing major decisions to be made at the unit level. The patient care manager, food services manager, or operating room manager can work out problems collaboratively among their departments because they have the autonomy, authority, and responsibility to do so. By contrast, in a centralized organizational structure problems among the departments would have to go to the nurse executive and then back down to the department managers—a much less efficient and more costly procedure.

Also, in the interest of cost-containment, patient care managers can collaborate in the management of their units by sharing personnel, hiring new people into flexible hour cycles, and sharing resources where appropriate.

NURSES IN EXPANDED ROLES: THE COLLABORATIVE PLAYERS

The nurse in an expanded role is defined by various titles—clinical specialist, nurse clinician, clinical nurse, or nurse practitioner. All of these titles have unique characteristics, and in each nursing organization they vary. This lack of clarity forces one to choose a generic term for the nurse in an expanded role. Nurse clinician will be the term used in this discussion.

Nurse clinicians bring expert knowledge and skill to an environment for collaboration. They work throughout the organization modeling collaboration at the clinical level with other nurses, with physicians, with patient and family, and with community agencies. Nurse clinicians also model collaboration with the executive level as they participate on hospital-wide committees and special projects related to patient care. Nurse clinicians are prepared at the master's or doctoral degree level to design and carry out research, consult, educate, and give patient care and thus are seen as peers of many of the leadership people in the organization. With their specialization in clinical practice, e.g., neonatology or cardiovascular nursing, they are in a position to share their knowledge and skill in a collaborative way with specialized teams. This expanded role also allows the staff nurses to observe collaborative practice and gives them a person or role to emulate as they work on behalf of their patients. The expanded role is a critical position in establishing an environment for collaboration.

Pam (a nurse clinician) and Sue (a primary nurse) were working with Billy, who was admitted with a diagnosis of child abuse. Both nurses had worked with many such children before. However, Pam sensed that Billy had many needs that other abused children did not demonstrate. She was used to collaborating with many team members and suggested that a psychiatric consult would be helpful to them as nurses and to Billy as the patient. The primary nurse disagreed with Pam's thinking. Her nursing assessment and intervention was adequate. Pam persisted, and a psychiatrist began working with Billy and the staff. Later the primary nurse realized that the collaborative effort in this case was effective and beneficial to both the patient and the staff.

Nurse clinicians are also pace setters for professional practice. They are constantly looking for new and better methods, reading the literature, attending conferences, talking with colleagues, and doing their own research to improve patient care. This group of nurses can also be influential in working with physicians in changing their attitudes for nursing generally. If a particular doctor has experienced a good collaborative relationship with a nurse clinician, he or she will tend to be more open to the ideas and the collaboration of other nurses within that organization. Of course the physicians are looking for credibility in expert knowledge and skill.

When the nurse executive is working in a collaborative mode and modeling executive traits, then that person will be supportive to the nurse in the expanded role or the nurse in the staff position working in a collaborative relationship. Administrative support would also be reflected in the fact that the nurse executive has hired nurse clinicians in appropriate numbers for the particular organization to be the role models for the staff and to work with other health care professionals on behalf of patient care. The nurse executive's support is also reflected by incorporating the nurse clinician into long-range planning committees, problem-solving activities, and general weekly or regular administrative meetings in which decisions for patient care are discussed and made. A nurse in an expanded role can be invaluable in creating a climate for collaboration, if the leadership is supportive and flexible. In one study of job satisfaction for clinical specialists, Shaefer defined administrative support as "aid given the clinician by nursing and hospital administrators and included advice, encouragement, and sanctions to her role as indicated by the salary she received, the authority vested in her, and the willingness of administrators to support her ideas and projects."[20]

Brown, in discussing the interdependence of nursing administrators and the clinical nurse specialist (CNS), says

> This is a useful, pragmatic definition, but it overlooks the collaborative aspect of support. Support is primarily an interpersonal process that takes place between the clinician and nursing or hospital administrators. Shaefer's definition implies that the clinician seeks, needs, or desires something from the administrative person. This is true: the CNS does need guidance, recognition, feedback, active acts of advocacy for her or his goals, and, at times, emo-

tional sustenance. The other reality of this relationship, however, is that the administrator is dependent on the nurse clinician in several ways. The administrator needs productivity from the CNS to meet departmental goals in patient care delivery; input and collaborative assistance in planning broadly for the department; and the vital clinical expertise and involvement that are at the heart of the CNS role. In fact, the relationship is an interdependent one; it should be viewed and operationalized as truly collegial and collaborative, rather than hierarchical. Even though the relationship has hierarchical aspects, they should be minimized in day-to-day dialogue. . . . It is extremely important, however, that this supportive style of leadership (participative management style, if you prefer) be utilized consistently, not just when it is convenient or when it is to the supervisor's advantage. Going back and forth between a collegial style and a hierarchical one can be confusing and frustrating to the CNS, since she or he never knows what the "style du jour" is.*

The qualities of a nurse who assumes this role are very specific. Preparation at the graduate level is basic, along with enough experience to bring a solid clinical knowledge base. Also, being a risk-taker is essential. To assess what is going on in a particular unit and see how it could be improved, then knowing step-by-step how to bring about that improvement and taking the risk to "stir up the waters" is a valued quality in a person in this role. This also requires assertiveness, speaking one's mind objectively, stating facts, and being able to get one's point of view across in a clear and direct manner without being too pushy or aggressive.

Another valued quality is the ability to do autonomous interventions, to be confident and knowledgeable enough to make decisions apart from other members of the health care team where appropriate and carry them out on behalf of the patient. This freedom is one of the rich rewards of a collaborative environment. Where mutual respect and give-and-take is active on a team, the nurse has freedom to make nursing decisions on behalf of the patient without checking everything out with the physician or other team members.

The physician has the opportunity to become more expressive in the process of this new relationship. Also, as nurses increasingly

---

*Reprinted from Sarah Jo Brown, "Administrative Support," in *The Clinical Nurse Specialist in Theory and Practice*, edited by Ann B. Hamric and Judy Spross, pp. 156–157, with permission of Grune & Stratton, Inc., © 1983.

exercise more accountability, the pressure upon physicians is lessened, as is their currently extensive legal vulnerability. Most significantly, though, it is likely that the physician will learn to appreciate the joys of colleagueship as he works with competent nurses.

For the nurse, the experience of a collaborative relationship with physicians and other health care providers has meant coming into her own. She finds a new fulfillment in her practice, in her ability to achieve competence in the application of the nursing process, and in being able to evaluate its efficaciousness. The colleagueship with other health care providers is personally rewarding and professionally reaffirming.[21]

If one is a risk-taker, is assertive, and performs autonomous interventions for patients and families, one must be accountable for those actions. This accountability is very important in the collaborative arena in that other health care members need to know the reasons why and the process used to come to certain decisions. The nurse in an expanded role can be dynamic in an organization as it moves toward greater collaboration with all members of the health care team.

The way nurse clinicians are placed in an organization is also important in establishing an environment for collaboration. Staff positions probably enable them to model collaboration for staff nurses in a better way than a line position would. According to French and Raven, there are five types of power: (1) legitimate power, which stems from one's position within the organization; (2) reverent power, which stems from the personality of the individual; (3) reward power, which stems from one's ability to dispense rewards; (4) coercive power, which stems from one's ability to coerce; and (5) expert power, which stems from one's experience in a given area.[22] (See also French and Raven, pp. 271–272.) The advocates of staff positions believe that nurse clinicians can accomplish their objectives by using expert and reverent power. This keeps the nurse clinician out of the traditional hierarchical structure and keeps the nurse clinician "truly professional." One of the problems with this is that the nurse clinician as a consultant trying to influence patient care may have excellent ideas and expert knowledge, but people holding line positions are the ones who carry out the recommendations. A head nurse, or patient care manager, for instance, may choose not to collaborate with the nurse clinician.

A long-term patient on a unit had no contact with his two siblings for four months. This occurred because the family lived a great distance from the hospital, and transportation could be arranged only if the siblings were allowed to spend the night. Money was not available to permit housing outside the hospital. Although the hospital visiting policy allowed sibling visiting for long-term patients, the patient care manager would not allow the overnight visit because it was not referred to in the visiting policy.

No amount of persuasion by the nurse clinician could get the patient care manager to change her decision. Finally, the mother informed the nurse clinician that she was removing her son from the hospital against medical advice so that the patient and siblings could have contact.

The mother's threat was conveyed to the patient care manager, and the visit was allowed to occur. In this case the mother used her power!

The nurse clinician in a staff position has freedom within the organization to work with patients on various units, both within the hospital and in the outpatient area, providing continuity of care. There is also flexibility of time; if home visits or working with community agencies on behalf of the patient is necessary, the nurse clinician is free to carry out these activities. Also, there is freedom to work on committees and change projects that benefit the entire patient care area, not just one small group of patients located in one geographic area of the hospital.

> The scope of responsibility for each CNS should be kept small enough to allow considerable involvement in the activities of her or his assigned units. If the nurse clinician is a member of a consultative or multidisciplinary care team, the case load must be of a size that allows time for follow-through, literature review, and some extemporaneous contact with staff. This limiting of the scope of responsibility may mean that some units or patient groups do not have the benefit of CNS influence; this is unfortunate, and further positions should be sought, but it is a sounder approach than stretching the CNS's scope of responsibility just so that each unit or each patient group is "covered" by CNS service. In overextending the CNS's scope of responsibility, the credibility of the role is decreased, its impact is diluted, and the frustrations of the CNS are heightened. The staff will bring problems to the CNS or the specialist will see them her- or himself, but the CNS will be unable to truly address the problems because of conflicting demands for her or his time. This lack of ability to respond to staff requests and the small amount of time the specialist is available to the staff can seriously undermine the credibility and effectiveness of the role.[23]

The expanded role of the nurse clinician enables an organization to model collaboration on a daily, unit-by-unit basis. Nurse clinicians collaborate with the patient and family in how nursing care is given and when, in health teaching, and in discharge planning. They also collaborate with the physicians and primary nurse to accomplish the goals set by the health care team. They collaborate with social workers, dietitians, and home health care agencies to ensure followup and continuity of care after hospitalization.

An organization with an adequate number of nurse clinicians is structured for collaboration. If the concept of collaboration is valued, it can be accomplished over time.

PRIMARY NURSES: THE COLLABORATIVE PLAYERS

Primary nursing was a direct reaction to the inability of the team system to deliver nursing care that was coordinated, individualized and comprehensive. Instead of fragmented care, the case method is used. Instead of complex channels of communications, simple direct patterns are used. Instead of shared responsibility, individual responsibility is clearly allocated.[24]

Decentralized decision making is the best foundation for primary nursing. It means simply the granting of decision-making authority to those at the level of action who are in the best position to judge the adequacy and efficacy of the decisions they make (see Chapter 1). It recognizes the value of individuals within all levels, putting them in control of their own actions. In primary nursing, decentralization means bringing decision making back to the bedside. Nurses need and are given responsibility for the nursing care received by a patient around the clock, seven days a week. They are authorized to direct the action of the other nurses who care for their patients when they are not there, which presupposes their respect and trust as essential ingredients in their interpersonal relationships. Therefore, mechanisms of accountability need to be established so that the quality of their decisions as primary nurses can be examined to determine whether or not good clinical judgment is being used.

Members of the management team best facilitate the implementation of primary nursing by adopting an attitude of support without pressure, as most nurses want to take good care of their patients. Support without pressure is an important mindset for the management team. Primary nursing cannot be implemented well by management edict. It must be implemented by the unit staff, those involved in delivering the care. A positive belief about nurses' commitment to giving good patient care also results in reasonable tolerance toward human error. A serious impediment to successful implementation of primary nursing is staff nurses' fear of confrontation with the realization that their names must go on the front of the chart. Management teams must discuss with the staff their attitudes toward making a mistake and actively educate for collaboration as part of the implementation of primary nursing.

> Contrary to popular belief, the autonomy often referred to in primary nursing was never meant to mean "alone." Autonomy is self directedness in which the individuals make multiple decisions about where to put time and energy. This is done within the context of broad expectation and individual expectation, "professional ideals." At this phase of autonomy, the nurse manager is a powerful influence. The nurse manager is needed to define an overall structure within which primary nurses can be self-directed and will request the nurse manager's knowledge or support when necessary. The nurse manager sets a crucial example for attitudes toward authority and responsibility. As primary nurses watch the way a nurse manager handles authority and responsibility for a nursing staff every day, week and month, they learn a powerful lesson about how such functions are handled.[25]

To be held accountable for their work with primary patients, primary nurses must be evaluated on the way they carry out each of their responsibilities. The evaluation should stimulate personal introspection, which allows them to grow in their abilities, attitudes, and actions. Only with feedback can primary nurses be fairly held accountable for the outcomes of these actions. Thus, accountability alone is necessary but not sufficient for primary nursing practice. The nurse manager needs to treat evaluations of primary nurses as an important aspect of managing toward accountability. Evaluations can also be used as tools for discussion about a primary nurse's career.

Terry was an average primary nurse who gave her patients excellent physical care, offered emotional support, and taught and interpreted activities related to daily inpatient care. However, her view of the patient was limited to current in-the-hospital happenings. As her patient care manager and nurse clinician reviewed care plans and documentation, the growing edge became very clear. A conference was set up and aspects of teaching and discharge planning were discussed for Terry's primary patients. Later this was followed up and reinforced. Affirmation was given as Terry demonstrated growth in response to the counseling of the patient care manager and nurse clinician. Over time, Terry grew into an excellent primary nurse, giving comprehensive care to her patients and actively collaborating with all members of the health care team. Due to the ongoing evaluation of each patient care plan, this primary nurse grew in her nursing practice.

When primary nursing is implemented, the stage is set for collaboration among the nurse, the patient, and the family; between nurse and nurse; between physician and nurse; between other health care personnel and the nurse. The nurses at the bedside interacting with the patient during many of the most significant happenings of the patient's hospitalization (and understanding the significance of those happenings to the patient) then can share this perspective with other members of the health care team to develop a plan of care. This communication and compromise that goes on among the health care team members promotes collaborative practice.

Collaboration can best be accomplished by patient care conferences where an interdisciplinary team sits down, and the physician, nurse, social worker, respiratory therapist, physical therapist, whoever is involved with the patient, share from their point of view and include the patient and family. Then new plans can be made and ongoing care given. In these conferences, the nurse has equal parity with all the other professions. The primary nurse's intimate knowledge of the patient enables him or her to individualize the care and to encourage the other team members to do the same. This collaborative effort promotes the nurse's self-actualization as a professional speaking on behalf of the patient, which not only provides quality care for the patient but is a morale booster for the individual nurse who feels that he or she is performing his or her role as a professional person.

A primary nurse collaborating with the health care team is illustrated by the following case study.

Brian P., age 11, was admitted with a diagnosis of AML, a serious form of leukemia. He was bright, verbal, dependent on his mother, and mildly hyperactive. Brian coped with hospitalization, exams, and some treatments; however, needles "spooked him," and he lost all control. One form of chemotherapy was ordered intrathecally, thus an LP needed to be performed each time this medication was administered. This procedure was difficult and painful for Brian, as his spine was abnormal and the spaces extremely close together, requiring several sticks before one could get into the proper space.

Brian's primary nurse worked to prepare him by explaining the procedure on his level. Coping behaviors were discussed, and a contract was made between the primary nurse and Brian. However, he could not tolerate the procedure and lost control, thrashing about and cursing the staff. His acting out behavior was so upsetting he increased his temperature, which was counterproductive.

The primary nurse initiated a meeting of all care givers—associate nurse, clinical nurse specialist, recreational therapist, social worker, and physician.

She presented a written summary of Brian's strengths and weaknesses, detailing especially well his psychological state and underlining the treatment goal of getting Brian into remission. The team members discussed various means to this end and how each would support the final decision.

Brian had been telling the primary nurse and his mother that he wanted to die; he planned his funeral and talked to his friends. He was refusing treatment. The primary nurse presented an alternative to the team suggestion—one drug be eliminated from treatment and the other two be continued. As the interdisciplinary team discussed further the wisdom of this suggestion, it was accepted. The physician discussed with the mother possible outcomes and had her sign necessary release papers. Brian continued his chemotherapy via intravenous route and went into remission. One year later he continues in remission. When he returns to the hospital he looks up his primary nurse with whom he has a special relationship.

Collaboration among primary nurses and other health care providers who work with primary patients is a hallmark of a professional milieu. Collaboration is part of patient advocacy as primary nurses become actively involved in daily discussions and decisions about patients. In one sense, primary nurses are the least prepared for collaboration of all the nursing personnel discussed so far. However, if the nurse executive sets the stage from the very top for collaboration, and the first-line managers model collaboration and are supportive of the staff nurse collaborating with other health team members, and the nurse clinicians in the organization are modeling collaboration as well as working with the primary nurses in collaborating with the health care team, primary nurses quickly learn the collaborative role. They not only collaborate with the health care team in terms of nurse to nurse, nurse to doctor, nurse to social worker, dietitian, or physical therapist, but they learn to collaborate with the patient and family in the best interests of that patient for care in the hospital and at home. Zander has summarized ten truths of collaborating for primary nursing that are succinct and helpful.[26]

Truth 1: Collaboration is easier when the desire for communication is abandoned. "Communicate" and "communication" have been overused as concepts to the point where they do not mean anything. They imply more than the exchange of information and cover a wide range of interrelationships between two or more individuals.

When the desire for communication is given up, primary nurses begin real collaboration. Collaboration requires primary nurses to decide ahead of time what and how facts and opinions will be presented to appropriate persons. When primary nurses put aside the desire for communication, they can collaborate more scientifically.

Truth 2: Collaboration is more effective in face-to-face contact than in medical charts or over the phone.

Personal contact is always best because body language adds honesty to the interaction. It is also easier to keep a person's attention. However, face-to-face discourse is less controlled than written messages.

Truth 3: Collaboration works best when personal issues are omitted and egos are put aside.

People can work together better if they do not feel that they are fighting for their esteem and their identity. Both parties must be able to save face and not lose pride in themselves because of a professional interaction.

Truth 4: Primary nurses can facilitate collaboration if they inform the physician of the pressures that are motivating them to collaborate.

This information should not be presented as an excuse or apology, but in an attempt to increase professional understanding.

Truth 5: Intimidation is the surest way to halt collaboration.

Intimidation is the social way of putting someone in their place, and it is the most prevalent disease in the hospital. Next to the patient, the nurse feels intimidated most often. Common signs of intimidation are power plays, orders written without planning or consulting nurses, and innuendos about the intellectual or scholastic deficits of nurses.

Truth 6: The most productive collaboration occurs before a crisis in the planning and replanning phases of patient care.

When physicians and primary nurses are not in the crunch of a crisis situation, collaboration is more likely and may even prevent crises. Frequent planning meetings between nurse and physician are useful, and physicians will learn that formal authority can be shared with nurses, thus lightening the burden of decision making.

Truth 7: Although ideal collaboration takes place as a style of planning, patient care situations require collaboration during crises.

In crisis situations, the guidelines developed by Bernstein et al. (1972), will be helpful to primary nurses:

1. Before contacting the doctor, do a conscientious job of assessing the patient's condition.
2. Then give him specific details.
3. When in doubt, call him. Don't wait, wondering.
4. Believe your own judgment, and don't be dissuaded if the doctor at first doubts it.
5. Use common sense in assessment, and try to correlate your findings.
6. Convey your belief that your role is important in patient care.
7. Keep your notes complete.
8. Don't be intimidated by the doctor. When it's vital, insist he listen.
9. Realize sometimes you may have to put yourself on the line; do it when you feel you should.
10. If you don't know the doctor's plans, ask him.
11. If you think his inaction is causing you problems, tell him.[27]

Truth 8: Not all problems and certainly not all feelings can be worked out through collaboration.

Sometimes primary nurses have to call in the nurse manager, supervisor, or the next in power above the physician with whom they are working. Primary nurses should be encouraged to use this avenue when certain problems arise, usually in emergency situations.

Truth 9: Not all difficulties in the nurse-physician relationship are based on female-male role stereotypes, but many are.

Although it is unproductive to blame all the faults in collaborative efforts on traditional male-female clashes, some female nurses tend to revert to behavior patterns which bog them down when they are dealing with male physicians.

Truth 10: New patterns of collaboration can be learned, though changes involve personal risk taking.

The nurse manager's values and style of collaboration greatly influence the motivation of primary nurses to broaden their approaches. Broaden is a better term to use than change, because as primary nurses find new techniques that work well, they gradually give up the less effective patterns. One good example of the gradual shift in the approach can be seen in the sequence:

  a. "There is nothing to be done about the situation" to
  b. "What can be done about the situation?" to
  c. "This is what can be done about the situation."[28]

Primary nursing sets the stage better than any other system of patient care delivery for collaborative practice. Primary nursing enables the nurse to self-actualize in the use of knowledge and skill with parity on the health care team. As the primary nurse grows in collaborative skill, job satisfaction and rewards from nursing practice will increase. This will keep highly skilled, well-qualified nurses at the bedside, doing what they do best.

QUESTIONS FOR THE FUTURE

The environment for collaboration has been discussed within the framework of an inpatient hospital setting. Organizational structure and various levels of personnel necessary for collaboration have been considered. The collaborative players at various levels of the organization have been defined and their interrelationships discussed.

Future questions to be considered are:

1. How can education for health care professionals better prepare them for collaborative practice?
2. What is the most effective way to educate for executive modeling in nursing administration?
3. How can we sustain a collaborative environment with the pressure of cost-containment?
4. What is the most effective way to document the cost-containment accomplished by collaboration?

NOTES

1. Abigail Trafford et al., "She's Come a Long Way—Or Has She?,"*U.S. News and World Report*, August 6, 1984, p. 44.

2. Ibid., p. 49.

3. Ibid., p. 51.

4. Belinda E. Puetz, *Networking for Nurses* (Rockville, Md.: Aspen Systems Corp., 1983).

5. Alexandra Symonds, "Emotional Conflicts of the Career Woman: Women in Medicine," *The American Journal of Psychoanalysis* 43, no. 1 (1983): 21–37.

6. Barbara J. Stevens, *The Nurse as Executive,* 2nd ed. (Rockville, Md.: Aspen Systems Corp., 1980), p. 193.

7. American Academy of Nursing, Task Force on Nursing Practice in Hospitals, *Magnet Hospitals: Attraction and Retention of Professional Nurses* (Kansas City, Mo.: American Nurses' Association, 1983).

8. Barbara J. Stevens, *The Nurse as Executive,* 2nd ed. (Rockville, Md.: Aspen Systems Corp., 1980), p. 199.

9. L.A. Bernhard and M. Walsh, *Leadership: The Key to Professionalization of Nursing* (St. Louis, Mo.: McGraw-Hill, Inc., 1981), p. 13.

10. Ibid., p. 14.

11. Ibid., p. 15.

12. Ibid., p. 18.

13. Marjorie A. Godfrey, "Job Satisfaction—Or Should That Be Dissatisfaction? How Nurses Feel about Nursing," Part One, *Nursing '78* 8, no. 4 (April 1978): 97.

14. Ibid., p. 98.

15. Ibid., p. 102.

16. Margretta M. Styles, *On Nursing: Toward a New Endowment* (St. Louis, Mo.: The C.V. Mosby Company, 1982), pp. 143–146.

17. T. Audean Duespohl, *Nursing in Transition* (Rockville, Md.: Aspen Systems Corp., 1983), p. 142.

18. *Webster's Third New International Dictionary,* Unabridged (Springfield, Mass.: Merriam-Webster, 1961).

19. T. Audean Duespohl, *Nursing in Transition* (Rockville, Md.: Aspen Systems Corp., 1983), p. 97.

20. J.A. Shaefer, "The Satisfied Clinician: Administrative Support Makes the Difference," *Journal of Nursing Administration* 3 (1973): 18.

21. Ingeborg G. Mauksch, "Nurse/Physician Collaboration: Nursing Practice Considerations," *The Journal of Nursing Administration,* June 1981, pp. 35–38.

22. J. French and B. Raven, "The Basis of Social Power," in *Studies in Social Power,* ed. D. Cartwright (Ann Arbor, Mich.: Institute of Social Research, University of Michigan, 1970).

23. Ann B. Hamric and Judy Spross, *The Clinical Nurse Specialist in Theory and Practice* (New York: Grune & Stratton, Inc., 1983), p. 162.

24. Marie Manthey, *The Practice of Primary Nursing* (Boston: Blackwell Scientific Publications, Inc.) 1980, p. 23.

25. Karen S. Zander, *Primary Nursing: Development and Management* (Rockville, Md.: Aspen Systems Corp., 1980), p. 39.

26. Ibid., pp. 216–221.

27. S. Bernstein, A. Hinton, and P. Taylor, "Trouble Communicating with Doctors," *Nursing '78* 2, no. 1 (January 1972): 33.

28. M. Menikheim, "Communication Patterns of Women and Nurses," in *Women in Stress: A Nursing Perspective*, eds. D. Kjervik and I. Martinson (New York: Appleton-Century-Crofts, 1979), p. 139.

SUGGESTED READINGS

Aiken, Linda H. *Nursing in the 1980's—Crisis, Opportunities, Challenges.* Philadelphia: L.B. Lippincott, 1983.

American Nurses' Association. *Nursing—A Social Policy Statement.* Kansas City, Mo.: American Nurses' Association, 1980.

Arnat and Huckabay. *Nursing Administration: Theory for Practice With a Systems Approach.* St. Louis: The C. V. Mosby Company, 1975.

Bernstein, S.; Hinton, A.; and Taylor, P. "Trouble with Communicating with Doctors." *Nursing '72* 2 (January 1972): 30–36.

Blake, Patricia. "The Clinical Specialist as Nurse Consultant." *Journal of Nursing Administration,* December 1977, pp. 33–36.

Chaska, Norma L. *The Nursing Profession: A Time to Speak.* St. Louis, Mo.: McGraw-Hill, Inc., 1983.

Devereux, Pamela McNutt. "Essential Elements of Nurse-Physician Collaboration," *The Journal of Nursing Administration* (May 1981): 19–23.

Devereux, Pamela McNutt. "Nurse/Physician Collaboration: Nursing Practice Considerations." *The Journal of Nursing Administration,* September, 1981, pp. 37–39.

Douglass, Laura Mae, and Bevis, Em Olivia. *Nursing Leadership in Action: Principles and Application to Staff Situations.* 2nd. ed. St. Louis, Mo.: The C.V. Mosby Company, 1974.

Fairbanks, Jane E. *Primary Nursing: More Data.* Rockville, Md.: Aspen Systems Corp., 1981, pp. 51–62.

Grissum, Marlene, and Spengler, Carol. *Womanpower and Health Care.* Boston, Mass.: Little Brown and Co., 1976.

Hamric, Ann B., and Spross, Judy. *The Clinical Nurse Specialist In Theory and Practice.* New York: Grune & Stratton, Inc., 1983.

Kramer, Marlene. *Reality Shock: Why Nurses Leave Nursing.* St. Louis, Mo.: The C. V. Mosby Company, 1974.

Marrana, Gwen A.; Schlegal, Margaret W.; and Bevis, Em O. *Primary Nursing: A Model for Individualized Care.* St. Louis, Mo.: The C.V. Mosby Company, 1974.

McGreevy, Mary E., and Coates, Mary R. "Primary Nursing Implementation Using the Project Nurse and the Nursing Framework." *The Journal of Nursing Administration,* February 1980, pp. 9–15.

Meisenhelder, Janice Bell. "Networking and Nursing." *Image* 14, no. 3 (October 1982): 77–80.

Menikheim, M. "Communication Patterns of Women and Nurses," in *Women in Stress: A Nursing Perspective.* Edited by D. Kjervik and I. Martinson. New York: Appleton-Century-Crofts, 1979.

National Joint Practice Commission. *Guidelines for Establishing Joint or Collaborative Practice in Hospitals.* Chicago, Ill.: Neely Printing Company, 1981.

Shaefer, J.A. "The Satisfied Clinician: Administrative Support Makes the Difference." *Journal of Nursing Administration* 3 (1973): 17–20.

Van Servellen, Gwen Marram. "Evaluating the Impact of Primary Nursing: Outcomes." *Nursing Dimensions,* Winter 1980, pp. 48–50.

Chapter 4

Attributes of the Professional Collaborator

Mary Mills Redman, R.N., M.S.N.

INTRODUCTION

This chapter encompasses a variety of concepts important to collaboration and professionalism, especially as applied to nursing. The model used for discussion is the discipline of nursing, but applications can be made to many other disciplines. The chapter will be presented in two parts.

The first part is a discussion of how good collaborative skills can become an attribute that influences all of the domain of nursing. Collaboration is seen as an umbrella that affects every aspect of our emergence as a profession.

The second part discusses the development of nursing as a profession, taking the view that nursing is a profession that is maturing and moving forward on the professional continuum. This includes emphasis on the important part that our individual beliefs about nursing and our beliefs about ourselves plays in our own professional development. This leads to discussion about our practice, which focuses on nursing behaviors and activities and their importance to professionalism. Next, current dilemmas within the whole of nursing are considered along with the need to establish goals that we can approach in unison instead of in conflict. The final discussion is based on the importance that the social policy statement has in helping nurses clearly define themselves both inwardly as nurses and outwardly as an important part of the whole of nursing.

A summary ties the chapter parts together and draws conclusions about the important role that finely tuned collaborative efforts can play in our advancement along the professional continuum.

Concerning the professional continuum, a discipline is viewed as being either more or less professional. Over time, the discipline can move in either direction on the continuum. The factors that influence forward movement are a sense of professionalism in individual members, the establishment of practice behaviors and activities that are considered important to professionalism, and a sense of unity in establishing and meeting organizational goals important to the profession. Each of these factors comes under the umbrella of collaboration, which literally means "working together"; the only way that we can become a unified profession is to work together and help each other.

COLLABORATION AS AN ATTRIBUTE

As we all know, our behavior depends on beliefs, attitude, personality, motives, learning, perception, maturity and aging, innate ability, and temporary conditions. Even more complicating is the fact that these characteristics influence and interact with each other. The way in which we work together, or collaborate, is a complex behavior determined by the interaction of these characteristics within each of us and the characteristics of those with whom we collaborate.

Of all these characteristics, our innate ability, beliefs, attitudes, and personality traits are the most constant. As we learn about ourselves, we learn how these factors influence our attempts to interact and collaborate with others. Through self-awareness and communication with others, we begin to understand that differences in beliefs, attitudes, and personality influence our ability to collaborate, and we learn how we can use these personal characteristics to our advantage instead of allowing them to become detrimental. For instance, if I as a nurse believe that all families should care for their terminally ill family members at home when physical care requirements make that possible, I need to acknowledge that opinion as a personal value and belief. I need also to realize the effects this belief could have in collaborating with other health team members about discharge planning and in collaborating with the family whose needs might best be met through the use of hospice care for their dying family member. My task here is to understand that my beliefs under these circumstances are only one way of perceiving this situation, that my role as a nurse collaborator is to explore with the family and other health team members the options available for caring for the sick family member, and then to be supportive of their decision.

Personality is another important characteristic influencing our ability to collaborate effectively. We need to be conscious of our own personality traits as well as the traits of others. For example, if we have a predominantly aggressive rather than a passive trait, we need to learn how to modify this trait so it becomes an asset to our collaborative efforts.

The characteristics of behaviors that are changing are our motives, maturity, and perception. Other changing conditions that are temporary include personal fatigue, temperature, environmental stress, and so on, and we need to be aware of how they affect our collaborative behavior. A motive can be either an impulse or an incentive that causes one to take action. In developing good collaborative skills, we need to be sure that our actions are based on important and appropriate incentives rather than on an inappropriate impulse. We need to gather background information, use the problem-solving process, and think about our actions before we get involved. We need to answer these questions positively: What is my role in this situation? Why is my involvement important? Perception, or the way in which we receive, organize, and interpret incoming information, is what helps us to answer these questions and what helps us to interact in a collaborative situation and to adjust to the varying demands of working together. It is extremely important to realize that each of us perceives incoming information in our own way, and we may have differences in the way we perceive the same information. Understanding this process requires maturity and a lack of self-centeredness.

Learning is a unique determinant of behavior and of our collaboration skills. Many behavioral scientists believe that we can learn only through active experience; others believe we can learn through example. In the health care arena there are many opportunities both to experience and to watch others collaborate. The maturity that we develop through experience and learning is invaluable in our collaborative efforts. Development and improvement of our communication skills and knowledge of group behavior has been explored in detail in Chapter 1. A practical way for us to learn about how we look, literally, when we collaborate is to use videotaping. This supplies us with immediate feedback about our behavior, and with the constructive feedback of others we can evaluate our collaboration abilities: did we come to the situation with adequate and appropriate knowledge, did we communicate effectively, did we exhibit good listening skills? With the use of mock collaboration situations and role playing, we can also learn about the importance of timing, overall stress, motives, personality traits, personal appearance, and so on. This learning process can be beneficial to virtually all of the collaborative behavior that occurs within our organization.

A substantial amount of behavioral research suggests that the most important sources of influence on how we are perceived by others involved in collaboration are our knowledge of our subject and situation, our motives, and personality. Factors that secondarily influence the attention given to us by others are our timing of communication efforts, physical appearance, and temporary conditions.

All behavior in the work setting influences our collaboration efforts. How we conduct ourselves at all times, our telephone etiquette, our casual and personal conversations, and our work under high and low stress conditions are all influential to others and how they perceive us as being worthy of collaboration. (I hope the reader will keep in mind these factors, so important to making collaboration an attribute, as the discussion of professionalism unfolds.)

THE DEVELOPMENT OF NURSING AS A PROFESSION

Over the past two decades, nurses have become increasingly intrigued with nursing as a profession. We have discussed and written extensively about how nursing fits into the professional arena. Most of the ways in which nurses have approached the issue have been to fit nursing into the traditional requirements initiated by Abraham Flexner in 1915. He proposed that a profession is characterized by activities that are intellectual in nature based on scientific inquiry, is used for unselfish purposes that serve society, can be taught and learned only through extensive educational preparation, and has internal control over its organization and members.[1] Others have expanded these criteria to include the following: has independent responsibilities, has collegiality with other services, has a code of ethics, and gives the community power to determine the need for the service, define how it operates, and accord it prestige.

To complicate matters, the word "professional" is also used prevalently in conjunction with anyone who has special training and receives payment for a job. However, the use of the word strictly as an adjective, such as professional carpenter, photographer, or painter, does not provoke a major controversy because the connotation is clearly different from that of the traditional professions. Identification of a group of individuals who make up a discipline that serves society's essential needs, such as health, education, or social, however, does provoke the "professional versus paraprofessional versus nonprofessional" controversy. Nursing does fit into this category.

Regarding professionalism, nurses today continue to struggle with some of the same questions Flexner had. The philosophical nature of these questions plays an important role in helping each of us generate our own thoughts and ideas about nursing as a profession. Margretta Styles views the issue of professionalism as an individual task in which our own self-identity and individual beliefs about the nature of nursing are the seeds that will endow nursing as a profession.[2] Many sociologists, historians, and nurses have viewed professionalism as a continuum along which the service-oriented disciplines may advance. In reconsidering the traditional definition, Styles believes nursing scores moderately well on all criteria, with our deficits being a strong theory base and self-control.[3] Stuart has called the traditional criteria a "theoretical and idealistic checklist approach," which is not met by any discipline in the purest sense.[4] One criterion states that the service orientation be totally unselfish. Many in the traditional professions currently practice at a substantial mercenary level. Nursing meets this criterion as well as any of the professions, continuing to work for the welfare of others despite relatively low monetary gains.

My view of nursing as a profession is that it is a discipline that is advancing along the professional continuum. In Flexner's original proposal is a statement in which he stressed, "what matters most is a professional spirit," that strong sense of altruism or desire to help others in need.[1] While this idea of "professional spirit" has an animating quality, I believe it is our strong desire to help others who cannot care totally for themselves that provides nursing with a solid place on the professional continuum. In order to move forward in our professional pursuit, we need to examine our own nursing self-identity, behaviors important to professional practice, and the composite goals of nursing as a profession. Collaboration in these areas will lead us to becoming unified and will allow nursing to move ahead as a profession.

OUR SELF-IDENTITY

In her 1982 publication, *On Nursing: Toward a New Endowment,* Margretta Styles has challenged each of us as individuals to take a look within ourselves: "I believe the seeds of professional reformation lie in the individual. . . . Let us compete to become the best we can be within ourselves . . . to accomplish the purposes we set out to do."[5] The focus of this document is on our individual character, our growth, progress, attitudes, values, and beliefs about ourselves and about nursing. Styles speaks of *professionhood* as the "characteristics of the individual" and of *professionalism* as denoting the "composite character of the profession."[6] She goes on to say that professionalism of nursing is directly dependent on the self-actualizing process, or professionhood of the individual members. Our individual growth and progress must be anchored in our belief about the essential nature and purpose of nursing.[7]

If we are secure in our beliefs about ourselves and the importance of nursing practice, our behaviors in related activities such as collaboration, documentation, and pursuit of knowledge will reflect these beliefs and influence our movement on the professional continuum. Styles has eloquently proposed a statement of beliefs about the nature and purpose of nursing:

1. I believe in nursing as an occupational force for social good, a force that, in the totality of its concern for all human health states and for

mankind's responses to health and environment, provides a distinct, unique, and vital perspective, value orientation, and service.

2. I believe in nursing as a professional discipline, requiring a sound education and research base grounded in its own science and in the variety of academic and professional disciplines with which it relates.

3. I believe in nursing as a clinical practice, employing particular physiological, psychosocial, physical, and technological means for human amelioration, sustenance, and comfort.

4. I believe in nursing as a humanistic field, in which the fullness, self-respect, self-determination, and humanity of the nurse engage the fullness, self-respect, self-determination, and humanity of the client.

5. I believe that nursing's maximum contribution for social betterment is dependent on:
   • the well-developed expertise of the nurse;
   • the understanding, appreciation, and acknowledgment of that expertise by the public;
   • the organizational legal, economic, and political arrangements that enable the full and proper expression of nursing values and expertise;
   • the ability of the profession to maintain unity within diversity.

6. I believe in myself and in my nursing colleagues:
   • in our responsibility to develop and dedicate our minds, bodies, and souls to the profession that we esteem and the people whom we serve;
   • in our right to be fulfilled, to be recognized, and to be rewarded as highly valued members of society.[8]

I propose here a challenge for each of us to read this inspirational work as part of renewing our commitment to nursing as an essential and important service to humanity. As we examine our beliefs and how they influence our practice, we would do ourselves a service to collaborate with other nurses and help each other strengthen our beliefs about ourselves as nurses. Since the inception of nursing, surveys and personal testimonies have repeatedly indicated that nurses believe that the most important aspect of nursing is caring, both in attitude and activity. As we support each other through collaboration, we exhibit both these qualities while strengthening our belief in ourselves, our peers, and our profession.

OUR PRACTICE

Two important recent advances in nursing practice to assure quality patient care have been the institution of primary nursing and nursing-focused quality assurance programs. Primary nursing has provided us with a tremendous opportunity to provide comprehensive patient care by allowing nurses to use their knowledge and make decisions for which they are accountable. It has also provided us with the opportunity for collaboration with the patient, with each other, with physicians, and with other members of the health care team. As we work together we enhance our ability to form collegial relationships and to be perceived by others as professionals.

Quality assurance programs have assisted us in looking systematically at nursing behaviors and activities that contribute to patient comfort and recovery, or to assist patients in caring for themselves. Quality assurance has included development of standards of care and the use of audits to determine if we are meeting our standards.

In a further attempt to determine what behaviors and activities nurses perform in practice and how important these are to their sense of professionalism, I and three other nursing colleagues developed a research survey to identify the comprehensive behaviors and activities that are practiced in nursing and their importance to professionalism. We decided to develop a survey instrument at St. Louis Children's Hospital in the interest of funding and convenience and with a conscious decision to focus on nurses who practice in the hospital setting, since this is where two out of three nurses are employed. A report of the nursing behaviors and activities research survey is included in Appendix 4-A. This represents beginning research and can be considered a pilot study since probability sampling was not used. No inferences can be made; however, the findings may have implications for all of us in our professional pursuit.

OUR GOALS

What are the goals of our profession? I believe a major goal is to become united in facing some important issues that challenge nursing today. We have just reviewed the current and potential strengths that lie in our patient care practice and our commitment. One could argue that these are all that really matter. These are what afforded us a place on the professional continuum; if we intend to move ahead, we must resolve our internal conflicts and rectify our deficits. We must resolve our stratified opinions regarding educational preparation, specialized nursing roles, theory development through research, membership in professional organizations, and the importance of collaboration.

The American Nurses' Association (ANA) has mandated that entry level into nursing practice will be the baccalaureate degree. This cannot possibly happen in practice until each of us agrees that college education is important to each of us as professionals and for the profession collectively. We must each do our part. Those of us who teach in baccalaureate programs need to offer assistance to those of us who teach in diploma programs so we can solve problems together in the process of transforming and combining these programs. A few schools have made these provisions and are testimony to the fact that it can be done if we are committed and collaborate with each other. Associate degree programs need to make provisions for easy transition to the universities, and those who choose not to continue toward the baccalaureate degree would practice nonprofessional nursing of a practical nature.

These ideas are not new and are not intended to diminish those who are currently practicing registered nurses with diploma and associate degrees. However, these individuals need to take responsibility in understanding the need for baccalaureate education as entry level into nursing practice as essential if nursing is to progress along the professional continuum. These nurses must also take responsibility for careful evaluation of their own educational needs depending on their own career goals and life circumstances, and all professional nurses should make this a continuing priority. Establishing the baccalaureate degree as entry level into practice will also raise the quality of applicants into our profession and influence our gains toward professionalization.

Another goal of our profession is to continue to ground our practice in research-based theory construction. We must continue with the use of the scientific method so we can support the nursing actions used to ameliorate patient problems. In her article on the professionalization of nursing, Stuart has proposed the emergence of a "researcher-theoretician" who addresses full-time the problem of scientific investigation and theory construction and who collaborates with other nurses across the country in these roles.[9] As individual professional nurses, we need to be supportive of these essential nursing roles so we can defend our professional standards.

A third goal of nursing is to increase political involvement, which will keep laws current, protecting the scope of nursing practice. We are each responsible for being conscious of national political issues and practicing our citizenship rights as well as being current on nursing practice laws and health-related issues.

A fourth goal of nursing is to become united through our professional organization. Increased membership and backing for individual nurses would allow the ANA more authority both within nursing and with other health professions. We each need to commit ourselves to making our professional organization work for us and become a building block in our professionalization.

Our ability to develop skills for collaboration is essential if we are ever to develop unity in reaching our professional goals. Collaboration is the piece that will tie us together as well as provide cohesiveness among our individual nursing identities, our practice, and our collective goals.

SOCIAL POLICY STATEMENT

The social policy statement of the ANA is a document that needs to be more widely used by most of us. It was intended "for use by nurses in achieving a fresh perspective on their practice, in helping the professional move forward at a speed consistent with soundness and based on the achievements already attained, and in giving society a current view of the nature of nursing practice."[10] This statement explains nursing's contribution to health care, and we should take advantage of using it. The social policy statement defines nursing as follows: A human concern, condition, event, need, or limitation to which nurses apply theory following assessment. Nurses decide what actions to take based on their assessment and knowledge of theory. The effects of nursing actions are evaluated in relation to the original human phenomenon.[11] This is the nature of nursing, an essential segment of meeting society's health care needs.

The social policy statement also considers other defining characteristics of nursing, such as:

- boundaries: defined by society's changing needs;
- intersections: missions and goals that are shared with other health professionals;
- care: the caring phenomena described previously are the core of nursing and what it offers society; this is highlighted by our ability to assess and arrive at treatment choices in nursing diagnosis;
- dimensions: further dimensions of nursing practice such as philosophy, ethics, behavior, commitment, specialization, generalization, interpersonal relationship skills, etc.[12]

Society may own our profession, but we, as individual nurses, own a part of what nursing is. We must continue to value ourselves and our *practice* as we move ahead in the health care arena. We also own our own behavior, and we must wake up to the fact that for nursing to advance on the professional continuum, we will run into conflict and we will have competition. We can come out ahead only if we develop our communication and collaboration skills so that our conflictive position becomes a challenge instead of a thorn.

CONCLUSION

Our ability to collaborate is important to us as individual nurses and to nursing as a profession. As individuals with refined collaboration skills we gain respect and are able to practice patient care of the highest quality. Collaboration with our nursing colleagues will help us understand each other and will provide support for our beliefs about the essential nature of nursing. Our practice is based on these beliefs, and our level of practice provides a major contribution to our professionalization. Collaboration is certainly the key to taking a unified approach to the goals of college level education, increase in ANA membership, political involvement, and so on. As we communicate with each other on a personal level and try to understand each other, we will truly be working together. Each of us must keep in mind that change takes time. We are closer to attaining professionhood as individual nurses than we've ever been before.

Our nursing beliefs (identity) lead to professionhood. Both the professionhood of our members and a unified approach to the goals discussed lead to professionalism.

NOTES

1. Abraham Flexner, "Is Social Work a Profession?," in *Proceedings of the National Conference of Charities and Corrections* (Chicago: Hildemann Printing Co., 1915), pp. 516–590.

2. Margretta M. Styles, *On Nursing: Toward a New Endowment* (St. Louis, Mo.: C.V. Mosby Co., 1982).

3. Ibid., pp. 44–45.

4. Gail Stuart, "How Professionalized is Nursing?," *Image: The Journal of Nursing Scholarship* 13 (1981), p. 18.

5. Margretta M. Styles, *On Nursing: Toward a New Endowment* (St. Louis, Mo.: C.V. Mosby Co., 1982), p. 57.

6. Ibid., p. 8.

7. Ibid., pp. 84–85.

8. Ibid., p. 61.

9. Gail Stuart, "How Professionalized is Nursing?," *Image: The Journal of Nursing Scholarship* 13 (1981).

10. American Nurses' Association, *A Social Policy Statement* (Kansas City, Mo.: ANA, 1980), p. 2.

11. Ibid., pp. 9–15.

12. Ibid., pp. 16–20.

SUGGESTED READINGS

American Nurses' Association. *A Social Policy Statement.* Kansas City, Mo.: ANA, 1980.

Anderson, R., and Carter, I. *Human Behavior in the Social Environment.* New York: Aldine Publishing Co., 1978, pp. 8–12.

Bandura, A. *Social Learning Theory.* New York: General Learning Press, 1971.

Cleland, Virginia. "The Professional Model." *American Journal of Nursing* 75 (1975): 288–292.

Flexner, A. "Is Social Work a Profession?," in *Proceedings of the National Conference of Charities and Corrections.* Chicago: Hildemann Printing Co., 1915, pp. 516–590.

Friedson, E. *Profession of Medicine.* New York: Dodd, Mead and Co., 1970.

Gamer, M. "The Ideology of Professionalism." *Nursing Outlook* 26 (1978): 51–55.

Gelin, A., and Duconus, A. *The Interdisciplinary Team.* Rockville, Md.: Aspen Systems Corp., 1981, pp. 39–59.

Goode, W. "The Librarian: From Occupation to Profession." *The Library Quarterly* 31 (1961): 306–318.

Goode, W. "The Theoretical Limits of Professionalization," in *The Semi-Professions and Their Organization.* Edited by A. Etzioni. New York: The Free Press, 1969, p. 278.

Goode, W. "Encroachment, Charlatanism, and the Emerging Profession: Psychology, Sociology and Medicine." *American Sociological Review* 25 (1960): 902–914.

Greenwood, E. "Attributes of a Profession." *Social Work* 2 (1957): 44–45.

Jacox, Ada. "Collective Action: The Basis for Professionalism." *Supervisor Nurse,* Sept. 1980, 22–32.

Johnson, Dorothy. "Professional Practice and Specialization in Nursing." *Image* 2 (1968): 2–7.

Kellams, Samuel E. "Ideals of a Profession: The Care of Nursing." *Nursing Image* 9 (1977): 30–31.

Mirton, R. "The Search for Professional Status." *American Journal of Nursing* 60 (1960): 662.

Moore, W. *The Professions: Roles and Rules.* New York: Russell Sage Foundation, 1974.

Porter, Lyman W. "Job Attitudes in Management." *Journal of Applied Psychology* 46 (1962): 375–384.

Purtilt, Ruth. *Health Professional/Patient Interaction.* Philadelphia: W.B. Saunders Co., 1978.

Stuart, Gail W. "How Professional is Nursing?" *Image* 13 (1981): 18–23.

Styles, Margretta M. *On Nursing: Toward a New Endowment.* St. Louis, Mo.: C.V. Mosby Co., 1982.

Styles, Margretta M. "Reflections on Collaboration and Unification." *Image: The Journal of Nursing Scholarship* 16, no. 1 (Winter 1984): 21–23.

Vollmer, H., and Mills, D. *Professionalization.* Englewood Cliffs, N.J.: Prentice-Hall, Inc., 1966.

Wilensky, H. L. "The Professionalization of Everyone?" *American Journal of Sociology* 70 (September 1964): 137–158.

Wolf, Margaret. "Group Stages: One View of the Development of the Nursing Profession." *Image* 9 (1977): 64–67.

PROFESSIONAL NURSING BEHAVIORS AND ACTIVITIES

STATEMENT OF THE PROBLEM

General discussion appears in the nursing literature regarding the professionalism of the discipline of nursing. In a review of the literature, however, none of the studies found addressed the issue in terms of behaviors and activities that would be essential to nursing practice if nursing is to gain professional status. Therefore, a need exists to generate this information from nurses who practice in patient care settings.

PURPOSE OF THE SURVEY RESEARCH

The purpose of this survey is to determine how registered nurses at St. Louis Children's Hospital define professional nursing in terms of behavior and activities. A survey questionnaire will be used for the population. These questions will be considered:

- How do registered nurses define professional nursing in terms of behavior and activities related to the scope of nursing practice?
- How important are these to professional nursing practice?
- How much are particular nursing behaviors practiced?
- Are there any differences in responses based upon the educational level of the registered nurse, membership in professional organizations, number of years nurses have been in practice, or habits used in reading professional journals?

REVIEW OF THE LITERATURE

The concepts of profession and professionalism have been defined, redefined, and argued for decades by historians, sociologists, members of "professional groups," etc. Required components of a discipline that give it professional status are:

- a sound theory base for practice,
- a body of knowledge specific to the discipline,
- development of specialized intellectual knowledge through extensive academic preparation,
- establishment of a mechanism for self-regulation and internal control, and
- having a service orientation that fulfills the vital needs of man.

Some of the ways in which nurses have approached the issue of professionalism in nursing practice have been:

- a comparison of nursing characteristics to the more traditional professional model with a proposal for viewing professionalism as a scale along which nursing may move if attention is paid to advanced education, construction of a sound theory base, specialization, etc.;[1]
- the use of collective bargaining toward development of a professional model for nursing practice;[2,3]
- nurse attitudes toward nursing practice and increased self-awareness of nurses as a basis for emerging as a profession;
- the importance of the work environment and its potential impact on the professionalism of nursing;
- the importance of internal beliefs about the nature and importance of nursing as a basis of the professionalism of nursing.[4]

As has been emphasized in other parts of this chapter, Margretta Styles has elaborated, in an extremely well-written document, on the ways in which professionalism has been described and judged by historians and on the social significance of the professions. The new endowment idea she gives to nursing refers to "our investment of a fresh perspective, natural capacity and power in ourselves—as nurses and as a profession."[5] She makes an important distinction between *professionhood,* meaning the individual characteristics of each member of the profession, and *professionalism,* which encompasses the composite character of the profession.[6] Her statement of emphasis is "the professionalism of nursing will be achieved only through the professionhood of its members."[7] Because the ideal of professionalism has been debated and criticized as being too limited and self-serving, Styles has suggested that we move beyond that approach. Her proposal for a model for nursing focuses on the character of its members and each individual's beliefs about the purpose and importance of nursing as part of the health care delivery system.[8] Styles proposes that our own personal self-actualization leads to the fullest expression as a nurse. However, she does not address professionhood in behavioral terms. The emphasis of this survey is to expand on Styles's strong base and incorporate behavioral components with the concepts.

METHODOLOGY

The survey questionnaire was developed and validated at St. Louis Children's Hospital. Initially, 10 percent of the registered nurses at St. Louis Children's Hospital were interviewed selectively to form a data base for development of the instrument. Data analysis of the interviews consisted of categorization of the responses and frequency distribution within the categories. The survey questionnaire was then developed and distributed to all registered nurses at St. Louis Children's Hospital (full- and part-time). Demographic data included number of years in nursing practice, current educational preparation, membership in nursing organizations, and habits of reading nursing journals. This was followed by 40 behavioral statements developed from the content of the interviews and the researcher's knowledge of nursing practice behaviors and behavioral trends in nursing. The respondent was then asked to consider each behavioral statement on two dimensions: (1) How much of this activity is there in my current nursing practice?; and (2) How important is this activity to professional nursing practice? (See Exhibit 1 for questionnaire and scoring of behavior and activity statements.) This scoring method was adopted from Porter's scale and used a 1–7 scale with 1 indicating a minimum amount of activity or importance to professional practice and 7 indicating a maximum amount of activity or importance of that activity to professionalism.[9]

Exhibit 1 Demographic Data

```
1. How many years have you practiced nursing? _____
2. What is your current educational preparation?
       _____ A.D.                        _____ B.S.N.
       _____ Diploma                     _____ Other
3. Membership in nursing organizations (check all please).
       _____ ANA                         _____ Critical Care
       _____ Sigma Theta Tau             _____ NLN
       _____ Other _____
4. Which nursing journals do you read regularly? (Please list.)
```

Exhibit 1 continued

QUESTIONNAIRE INSTRUCTIONS

Two scores are required for each item. Using a scale of 1–7 where *1 indicates minimum* and *7 indicates maximum*, please score each item in terms of:

1 = Never
2 = Occasionally
3 = Nearly half of the time
4 = Half of the time
5 = More than half of the time
6 = Almost always
7 = All of the time (always)

	How much do I do in my current nursing practice?	How important is this to professionalism?
5. Use of the complete nursing process: assessment, planning, intervention, evaluation.		
6. Care planned with the patient and family.		
7. Assessment of individual needs of patient and family.		
8. Nursing intervention individual-ized.		
9. Individualized teaching incorpo-rated into providing care.		
10. Discharge planning begun early in hospitalization.		
11. Relevant information communi-cated via documentation.		
12. Collaboration and coordination of care with other health team members.		
13. Priorities set daily in planning and giving patient care.		
14. Priorities set daily in organizing unit activities.		
15. Practice based on current knowl-edge of the patient's condition and changing treatment plans.		
16. Knowledge sought when presented with unfamiliar diagnoses or con-ditions.		

Exhibit 1 continued

	How much do I do in my current nursing practice?	How important is this to professionalism?
17. Accountable for nursing practice decisions made.		
18. Evaluation of care given by self and others and appropriate changes made.		
19. Consideration of physical, psychological, social, and spiritual aspects of patients/families.		
20. Nursing practice developed independent of medical directives.		
21. Patient and family input included in setting patient care priorities in meeting individualized patient needs.		
22. Priorities dictated by the patient and family needs.		
23. A balance maintained between task orientation and conceptual approaches to nursing practice.		
24. Problem-solving process used in setting priorities.		
25. Importance of maintaining open communication under stress recognized and reflected under stressful conditions.		
26. A supportive attitude to patient, family, and other staff maintained under stress.		
27. Importance of membership in professional organizations recognized.		
28. Professional literature related to nursing practice reviewed.		
29. Professional literature related to area of expertise reviewed.		
30. Participation in the institution's organizational activities.		

Exhibit 1 continued

	How much do I do in my current nursing practice?	How important is this to professionalism?
31. The need for ongoing continuing education in nursing recognized.		
32. The need for personal growth recognized.		
33. The role as an educator in nursing recognized.		
34. The role of broadening the base of nursing knowledge through research and publication recognized.		
35. New developments in nursing recognized and incorporated into nursing practice when appropriate.		
36. The development of nursing diagnosis understood.		
37. The nursing diagnosis model for nursing practice applied in practice.		
38. The concept of career ladder as a method of self-development in nursing practice understood.		
39. The primary nursing patient care delivery method used.		
40. A deliberate and continuous effort to evaluate practice made.		
41. Peer review sought in helping to evaluate practice.		
42. Patient/family outcome as a criterion for evaluating practice used.		
43. Knowledge put into practice.		
44. Practice decisions and changes based upon a continually updated knowledge base.		

Exhibit 1 continued

Please write a brief response to the next two questions.
45. What constitutes a "good day" for the professional nurse?
46. What are the drawbacks to being a professional nurse?
47. Are all registered nurses practicing professional nursing?
_____ Yes   _____ No
48. Is nursing a profession?
_____ Yes   _____ No
49. Why do/don't you think so?

QUESTIONNAIRE DISTRIBUTION, FOLLOWUP PROCEDURES, AND RESPONSE RATE

The personally delivered and personally collected method was used for questionnaire distribution. The questionnaires were put in the respondent's mail box in the hospital where each could not be personally contacted. When the respondents did not have a mail box, the questionnaire accompanied the respondent's paycheck. The return envelopes were addressed to the researchers, and each return envelope was coded for follow-up procedures. The nonrespondent group was contacted a second time. The response rate was 50 percent, with 156 of 311 questionnaires returned.

DATA ANALYSIS

Of those who responded to the survey (see Exhibit 2), 11 percent had been practicing nursing 2 years, 19 percent had practiced 2–3.99 years, 24 percent had practiced 4–7 years, and 46 percent had practiced more than 7 years. On the variable of current educational preparation, 14 percent had an associate degree, 36 percent had diplomas, 41 percent were B.S.N. prepared and 9 percent were M.S.N. prepared. Sixty-two percent did not belong to a professional organization and 38 percent belonged to one or more professional organizations. These numbers are consistent with the response (40 percent reported membership) to a recent questionnaire by Yeager and Kline, which addressed professional association membership of nurses and factors affecting the decision to join in 1983.[10] The last demographic variable addressed the nurse's habit of reading nursing journals regularly. Of these respondents, 35 percent reported that they did not read, while 65 percent read one or more nursing journals regularly.

Exhibit 2 Demographic Data

A. Years in nursing		2	2-3.99	4-7	7
		11%	19%	24%	46%
B. Current educational	A.D.	Diploma	B.S.N.	M.S.N.	
preparation	14%	36%	41%	9%	
C. Organizational	Do Not Belong		Belong to 1 or More		
membership	62%		38%		
D. Read nursing journals	Do Not Read		Read 1 or More		
	35%		65%		

Table 1 contains information regarding how the respondents scored each nursing behavior or activity in terms of its importance to professional nursing practice and how much each behavior/activity is incorporated into their current nursing practice. The behaviors/activities are presented in rank order with mean scores, standard deviation, and a correlation factor. The two behaviors that received the highest scores on importance to professionalism also were reported to be done most often in practice. These items were (1) accountable for nursing practice decisions made and (2) knowledge sought when presented with unfamiliar diagnoses and conditions. Generally items that addressed parts of the nursing process, maintenance of control under stressful conditions, updating one's patient knowledge, collaboration with colleagues and other professionals, and individualized care were felt to be most important to professional nursing practice. Items that scored next on importance to professionalism included documentation, continuing education in nursing, use of the complete nursing process, use of primary nursing method, and discharge planning. Items that received lowest scores on importance to professionalism included the need for nursing research and publications recognized, the importance of membership in professional organizations, and some trends in nursing, such as nursing diagnosis, career ladder, and peer review. The items that scored lowest on importance to professionalism also scored lowest on how much these activities were done in current nursing practice.

Items that had the most discrepancy (rank order difference greater than or less than 10) between importance to professionalism and done in practice were: (1) importance of maintaining open communication under stress recognized and reflected under stressful conditions, which ranked 4 on importance ($\bar{x} = 6.74$) and ranked 15 on done in practice ($\bar{x} = 5.52$); (2) relevant information communicated via documentation, which ranked 14 ($\bar{x} = 6.59$) and 24 ($\bar{x} = 5.12$) respectively; (3) the need for personal growth

Table 1

Column I: Behavior/activity statements are listed in rank order as reflected in the mean scores of the items on the dimension of importance to professionalism.

Column II/III: Mean and standard deviation for each behavior/activity statement on the dimension of importance to professionalism.

Column IV: Rank of each statement according to mean score reflecting how much the behavior/activity is done in practice.

Column V/VI: Mean and standard deviation for each behavior/activity statement on the dimension of how much is done in practice.

Column VII: Correlation of the importance of each behavior/activity with how much is done in practice.

I Item by Rank According to Importance to Professionalism	*II* Importance to Professionalism $\bar{x}$	*III* s	*IV* Rank According to How Much Done in Practice	*V* Do in practice $\bar{x}$	*VI* s	*VII* r
1. Accountable for nursing practice decisions made.	6.89	.33	1	6.43	1.32	.12
2. Knowledge sought when presented with unfamiliar diagnoses or conditions.	6.78	.43	2	6.00	1.36	.28
3. Assessment of individual needs of patient and family.	6.77	.72	5	5.90	1.55	.45
4. Importance of maintaining open communication under stress recognized and reflected under stressful conditions.	6.74	.56	15	5.52	1.35	.37
5. A supportive attitude to patient, family, and other staff maintained under stress.	6.73	.75	6	5.87	1.24	.49
6. Knowledge put into practice.	6.73	.52	3	5.97	1.33	.33
7. Practice based on current knowledge of the patient's condition and changing treatment plans.	6.70	.74	8	5.78	1.52	.45
8. Evaluation of care given by self and others and appropriate changes made.	6.70	.51	13	5.56	1.47	.28
9. Consideration of physical, psychological, social, and spiritual aspects of patients/families.	6.70	.54	17	5.44	1.41	.33
10. Nursing intervention individualized.	6.69	.74	9	5.72	1.52	.20
11. Collaboration and coordination of care with other health team members.	6.65	.83	18	5.41	1.53	.40

I Item by Rank According to Importance to Professionalism	*II* Importance to Professionalism x̄	*III* s	*IV* Rank According to How Much Done in Practice	*V* Do in practice x̄	*VI* s	*VII* r
12. Individualized teaching incorpo- rated into providing care.	6.65	.76	14	5.54	1.59	.22
13. Practice decisions and changes based upon a continually updated knowledge base.	6.64	.77	11	5.65	1.45	.18
14. Relevant information communi- cated via documentation.	6.59	.83	24	5.12	1.51	.33
15. The role as an educator in nursing recognized.	6.59	.75	7	5.81	1.49	.42
16. Priorities set daily in planning and giving patient care.	6.55	.88	10	5.70	1.65	.43
17. The need for personal growth recognized.	6.53	.87	4	5.94	1.38	.28
18. The need for ongoing continuing education in nursing recognized.	6.43	.90	12	5.57	1.68	.53
19. A deliberate and continuous effort to evaluate practice made.	6.42	.90	21	5.34	1.55	.20
20. Use of the complete nursing process: assessment, planning, intervention, evaluation.	6.39	1.15	19	5.40	1.53	.58
21. Care planned with the patient and family.	6.36	1.08	30	4.87	1.82	.48
22. Patient and family input included in setting patient care priorities in meeting individualized patient needs.	6.36	1.18	23	5.20	1.75	.52
23. Problem-solving process used in setting priorities.	6.32	1.04	20	5.36	1.46	.42
24. New developments in nursing rec- ognized and incorporated into nurs- ing practice when appropriate.	6.29	1.05	28	4.92	1.62	.44
25. The primary nursing patient care delivery method used.	6.20	1.29	16	5.48	1.78	.36
26. Patient/family outcome as a crite- rion for evaluating practice used.	6.17	1.20	27	4.94	1.80	.40
27. Professional literature related to area of expertise reviewed.	6.09	1.23	31	4.85	1.82	.61
28. Discharge planning begun early in hospitalization.	6.02	1.38	36	4.18	1.80	.47
29. Priorities set daily in organizing unit activities.	5.98	1.32	25	5.05	1.86	.53

Table 1 *continued*

I	*II*	*III*	*IV*	*V*	*VI*	*VII*
			Rank According to How Much			
Item by Rank According to Importance to Professionalism	*Importance to Professionalism*		*Done in Practice*	*Do in practice*		
	x̄	*s*		*x̄*	*s*	*r*
30. Priorities dictated by the patient and family needs.	5.96	1.40	26	5.05	1.81	.61
31. A balance maintained between task orientation and conceptual approaches to nursing.	5.95	1.38	32	4.74	1.69	.59
32. The development of nursing diagnosis understood.	5.95	1.54	22	5.28	1.70	.67
33. Peer review sought in helping to evaluate practice.	5.87	1.31	33	4.66	0.90	.58
34. Nursing practice developed independent of medical directives.	5.78	1.59	29	4.88	1.73	.73
35. Professional literature related to nursing practice reviewed.	5.76	1.44	34	4.37	1.89	.55
36. The role of broadening the base of nursing knowledge through research and publication recognized.	5.75	1.50	37	4.12	2.17	.52
37. The nursing diagnosis model for nursing practice applied in practice.	5.61	1.82	35	4.34	2.02	.58
38. The concept of career ladder as a method of self development in nursing practice understood.	5.09	2.02	38	4.08	2.09	.55
39. Participation in the institution's organizational activities.	5.04	1.73	39	3.94	1.94	.55
40. Importance of membership in professional organizations recognized.	4.66	1.95	40	3.28	2.02	.57

ranked 17 ($\bar{x} = 6.53$) and 4 ($\bar{x} = 5.94$), respectively; and (4) the development of nursing diagnosis understood ranked 32 ($\bar{x} = 5.95$) on importance to professionalism and 22 ($\bar{x} = 5.28$) on done in current practice. Of special interest is the item on primary nursing, which ranked much higher on done in current practice (rank = 16) than on importance to professionalism (rank = 25).

To determine if there were significant differences in mean scores for each item on both the "importance to professionalism" dimension and the "done in practice" dimension, F values were computed for each demographic category of number of years in nursing practice, educational preparation, organizational membership, and read nursing journals. When number of years in nursing was considered, there were no differences ($p < .05$) found on scoring of any items. Items that revealed the most differences (F values) across the other three demographic variables (education, organizational membership, journal reading) on both dimensions of importance to professionalism and done in practice are shown in Table 2.

To speculate on where the differences lie, we can look at the mean scores for the categorical variables: type of educational preparation, whether or not journals are read, and whether or not there is membership in professional organizations. Clearly, these particular items are both much more important to professionalism and are practiced more often by those nurses with higher educational preparation who read nursing journals regularly and who belong to professional organizations (See Tables 1, 3, and 4 for mean scores in each demographic category).

Table 2

Column 1: Importance to Professionalism
Column 2: Done in Practice

ITEM	*EDUCATION*		*JOURNALS*		PROFESSIONAL ORGANIZATIONS	
	1	2	1	2	1	2
Importance of membership in professional organizations recognized.	5.58***	8.10***	11.21***	22.11***	13.90***	46.34***
Professional literature related to nursing practice reviewed.	4.59***	4.31***	12.94***	45.74***	3 .86*	10.56***
Professional literature related to area of expertise reviewed.	3.25***	7.30***	19.88***	32.02***	4. 37**	11.52***
Participation in the institution's organizational activities.	2.77**	7.00***	3.08*	8.20***	2.33	6.15**
The role of broadening the base of nursing knowledge through research and publication recognized.	3.27**	1.13	14.92***	6.23***	5.94**	3.11*

***$p < .01$
**$p < .05$
*$p < .10$

Table 3

Computed F values for difference in item mean scores where:
Column A: Education (4 categories: A.D., Diploma, B.S.N., M.S.N.)
Column B: Journals (2 categories: Do Not Read, Read 1 or More);
Column C: Professional Organizations (2 categories: Do Not Belong, Belong to 1 or More)
Column D: Years in Practice (4 categories: 2 yrs., 2–3.99, 4–7, 7).
Column 1: Importance to Professionalism; Column 2: Done in Practice

Item	A Education		B Journals		C Professional Organizations		D Yrs in Nursing	
	1	2	1	2	1	2	1	2
Use of the complete nursing process: assessment, planning, intervention, evaluation.	4.55***	2.55	1.14	9.63***	0.12	0.07	1.43	0.62
Care planned with the patient and family.	0.75	1.48	0.17	2.55	0.55	0.14	0.07	1.42
Assessment of individual needs of patient and family.	0.44	0.06	0.91	5.81**	2.46	0.25	0.58	1.65
Nursing intervention individualized.	0.96	0.43	1.28	9.51****	0.18	0.06	0.21	0.76
Individualized teaching incorporated into providing care.	0.51	0.20	0.72	2.99*	1.05	0.91	0.89	1.34
Discharge planning begun early in hospitalization.	0.94	1.32	10.52***	11.12***	3.22*	0.27	2.57	1.15
Relevant information communicated via documentation.	0.17	0.31	7.28***	8.20***	0.62	1.83	0.23	0.47
Collaboration and coordination of care with other health team members.	1.95	0.40	1.44	2.91*	1.31	0.81	0.60	1.02
Priorities set daily in planning and giving patient care.	0.00	0.04	0.19	4.77**	4.81**	0.39	1.34	1.27
Priorities set daily in organizing unit activities.	0.32	3.03**	0.44	3.29*	0.04	0.10	0.18	0.51

Practice based on current knowledge of the patient's condition and changing treatment plans.	2.12*	0.80	0.14	6.42**	6.30**	0.43	0.48	0.21
Knowledge sought when presented with unfamiliar diagnoses or conditions.	0.71	0.47	1.13	16.36***	0.86	0.02	0.38	0.54
Accountable for nursing practice decisions made.	0.52	0.43	4.36**	3.05*	0.97	0.43	0.63	0.90
Evaluation of care given by self and others and appropriate changes made.	0.90	0.54	4.25**	7.07***	0.58	1.54	1.19	1.20
Consideration of physical, psychological, social, and spiritual aspects of patients/families.	1.99	0.64	0.21	4.02**	7.83***	0.11	1.26	1.14
Nursing practice developed independent of medical directives.	0.16	0.53	7.15***	5.79**	0.87	0.48	0.82	0.59
Patient and family input included in setting patient care priorities in meeting individualized patient needs.	0.69	0.06	0.68	1.53	2.45	0.87	0.58	0.16
Priorities dictated by the patient and family needs.	1.63	0.17	1.09	0.54	0.99	3.72*	0.12	0.42
A balance maintained between task orientation and conceptual approaches to nursing practice.	0.96	1.60	0.97	2.68	1.55	0.02	0.73	0.19
Problem-solving process used in setting priorities.	1.55	1.85	8.07***	11.68***	4.50**	1.92	0.38	0.15
Importance of maintaining open communication under stress recognized and reflected under stressful conditions.	0.93	1.01	2.17	4.09**	2.49	0.11	0.11	0.72
A supportive attitude to patient, family, and other staff maintained under stress.	0.27	1.10	0.04	1.28	2.80*	0.07	0.23	0.07

Table 3 continued

Item	Education		Journals		Professional Organizations		Yrs in Nursing	
	1	2	1	2	1	2	1	2
Importance of membership in professional organizations recognized.	5.58***	8.1***	11.21***	22.11***	13.90***	46.34***	0.44	0.89
Professional literature related to nursing practice reviewed.	4.59***	4.31***	12.94***	45.74***	3.86*	10.56***	2.22*	0.92
Professional literature related to area of expertise reviewed.	3.25**	7.3***	19.88***	32.02***	4.37**	11.52***	0.85	0.49
Participation in the institution's organizational activities.	2.77**	7.0***	3.08*	8.20***	2.33	6.15**	0.57	2.01
The need for ongoing continuing education in nursing recognized.	1.23	3.04**	10.14***	7.23***	0.73	0.89	0.82	0.60
The need for personal growth recognized.	1.00	1.08	7.44***	4.04**	0.02	0.07	1.81	0.47
The role as an educator in nursing recognized.	1.38	1.92	4.34**	7.47***	0.30	0.02	0.78	0.32
The role of broadening the base of nursing knowledge through research and publication recognized.	3.27**	1.13	14.92***	6.23***	5.94**	3.11*	0.29	0.91

New developments in nursing recognized and incorporated into nursing practice when appropriate.	0.84	0.90	7.09***	5.21**	0.09	0.00	0.48	0.40
The development of nursing diagnosis understood.	0.74	0.48	1.58	1.13	0.14	0.07	1.62	2.90**
The nursing diagnosis model for nursing practice applied in practice.	0.89	1.04	4.83**	0.90	0.57	0.23	1.43	2.33*
The concept of career ladder as a method of self-development in nursing practice understood.	1.41	1.77	0.14	4.13**	0.95	0.00	7.16***	1.73
The primary nursing patient care delivery method used.	1.31	0.16	0.27	1.33	0.88	0.00	1.51	2.07
A deliberate and continuous effort to evaluate practice made.	1.38	0.24	2.21	2.67	1.82	1.11	1.84	0.36
Peer review sought in helping to evaluate practice.	2.75**	0.54	0.83	0.02	0.02	1.62	0.51	0.76
Patient/family outcome as a criterion for evaluating practice used.	0.97	0.12	0.15	1.95	0.11	0.81	1.66	0.81
Knowledge put into practice.	0.14	0.37	7.37***	5.33	0.52	0.34	1.58	0.70
Practice decisions and changes based upon a continually updated knowledge base.	1.18	0.42	11.82***	5.88**	0.44	0.31	0.33	0.10

***$p < .01$
**$p < .05$
*$p < .10$

Table 4

Means and rank order on items scored showing a significant difference according to educational level of respondent on the importance to professionalism dimension.

| | | RANK ACCORDING TO EDUCATION | | | |
		A.D.	Diploma	B.S.N.	M.S.N.
1. $(F = 4.55)^{**}$ Use of complete nursing process.	$\bar{x}$	5.6	6.38	6.56	6.85
	Rank	32	20	17	3
2. $(F = 5.58)^{**}$ Importance of membership in professional organizations recognized.	$\bar{x}$	3.7	4.4	4.9	6.23
	Rank	40	40	40	36
3. $(F = 4.59)^{**}$ Professional literature related to nursing reviewed.	$\bar{x}$	4.9	5.57	6.02	6.53
	Rank	37	35	31	26
4. $(F = 3.25)^{*}$ Professional literature related to area of expertise reviewed.	$\bar{x}$	5.5	5.96	6.27	6.69
	Rank	33	30	25	16
5. $(F = 2.77)^{*}$ Participation in institution's organizational activities.	$\bar{x}$	4.55	4.7	5.24	6.0
	Rank	39	38	39	39
6. $(F = 3.27)^{*}$ The role of research and publication recognized.	$\bar{x}$	5.4	5.3	6.09	6.3
	Rank	35	37	29	33
7. $(F = 2.75)^{*}$ Peer review sought in evaluating practice.	$\bar{x}$	5.75	5.59	6.12	6.38
	Rank	31	34	28	31

$^{**}p. < .01$
$^{*}p. < .05$

In addition to the above items, as educational preparation increased, nurses believed that use of the *complete* nursing process was more important to professional nursing practice. It is also interesting that whether or not nurses read professional journals regularly indicates the most frequent differences in these behaviors scored as being important to professional nursing practice. Seventeen items were scored significantly higher ($p < .05$) on importance to professionalism by nurses who read nursing journals regularly compared with seven items scoring higher ($p < .05$) as the educational preparation level increased and seven items scoring higher ($p < .05$) by nurses who belong to professional organizations on importance to professionals. (See Tables 5 and 6.)

At the end of the survey, nurses were asked to designate whether they believe nursing is a profession and why they do or do not believe so. Twenty-five percent (39/156) of the respondents indicated that collaboration skills were essential to nurses who practice as professionals. Pertinent comments included:

Nurses who do not practice as professionals have poor collaboration skills which makes it impossible to learn the skills necessary to be professionals.

Collaboration with peers and physicians allows one to do a professional job.

We cannot possibly become a profession as long as we spend too much time stepping on each other instead of working together to help each other.

Nursing is a career. It is my profession.

. . . a very immature profession; still struggling to accept the need for academic credibility (B.S.N. as entry level).

Table 5 Journals

Means and rank order on items showing a significant difference according to whether or not journals are read on the importance to professionalism dimension.

		Do Not Read 35%	Read 1 or More 65%
1. ($F = 10.52$)** Discharge planning begun early in hospitalization.	$\bar{x}$	5.53	6.30
	Rank	32	26
2. ($F = 7.28$)** Relevant information communicated via documentation.	$\bar{x}$	6.35	6.72
	Rank	15	10
14. ($F = 4.36$)* Accountable for nursing practice decisions made.	$\bar{x}$	6.81	6.93
	Rank	1	1
15. ($F = 4.25$)* Evaluation of care given by self and others and changes made.	$\bar{x}$	6.59	6.78
	Rank	9	7

Table 5 *continued*

		Do Not Read 35%	Read 1 or More 65%
3. (F = 7.15)** Nursing practice developed independent of medical directives.	$\bar{x}$ Rank	5.31 34	6.04 33
4. (F = 8.07)** Problem-solving process used in setting priorities.	$\bar{x}$ Rank	5.98 25	6.49 20
5. (F = 11.21)** Importance of membership in professional organizations recognized.	$\bar{x}$ Rank	3.94 40	5.05 40
6. (F = 12.94)** Professional literature related to nursing practice reviewed.	$\bar{x}$ Rank	5.18 35	6.07 31
7. (F = 19.88)** Professional literature related to area of expertise reviewed.	$\bar{x}$ Rank	5.49 33	6.41 24
8. (F = 10.14)** Need for ongoing continuing education recognized.	$\bar{x}$ Rank	6.10 24	6.60 17
9. (F = 7.44)** Need for personal growth recognized.	$\bar{x}$ Rank	6.27 18	6.67 16
16. (F = 4.34)* The role as educator in nursing recognized.	$\bar{x}$ Rank	6.40 14	6.68 15
10. (F = 14.92)** The role of broadening the base of nursing knowledge through research and publication recognized.	$\bar{x}$ Rank	5.10 37	6.09 29
11. (F = 7.09)** New developments in nursing recognized and incorporated into nursing practice.	$\bar{x}$ Rank	5.98 26	6.47 21
17. (F = 4.83)* Nursing diagnosis model for nursing practice applied in practice.	$\bar{x}$ Rank	5.15 36	5.85 37

Table 5 *continued*		Do Not Read 35%	Read 1 or More 65%
12. $(F = 7.37)**$ Knowledge put into practice.	$\bar{x}$	6.57	6.82
	Rank	11	4
13. $(F = 11.82)**$ Practice decisions and changes based on updated knowledge base.	$\bar{x}$	6.35	6.80
	Rank	16	5

$**p < .01$
$*p < .05$

Table 6 Professional Organizations

Means and rank order on items showing a significant difference according to membership in professional organizations on the importance to professionalism dimension.

		Do Not Belong 62%	Belong to 1 or More 38%
3. $(F = 4.81)*$ Priorities set daily in planning and giving patient care.	$\bar{x}$	6.68	6.35
	Rank	12	21
4. $(F = 6.30)*$ Practice based on current knowledge of patient condition and treatment plan.	$\bar{x}$	6.83	6.51
	Rank	3	18
1. $(F = 7.83)**$ Consideration of physical, psychological, social, and spiritual aspects of patient/family.	$\bar{x}$	6.80	6.55
	Rank	6	14
5. $(F = 4.50)*$ Problem solving process used in setting priorities.	$\bar{x}$	6.17	6.55
	Rank	26	15
2. $(F = 13.90)**$ Importance of membership in professional organizations recognized.	$\bar{x}$	4.12	5.40
	Rank	40	38
6. $(F = 4.37)*$ Professional literature related to area of expertise reviewed.	$\bar{x}$	5.92	5.36
	Rank	29	20
7. $(F = 5.94)*$ The role of broadening the base of nursing knowledge through research and publication recognized.	$\bar{x}$	5.51	6.13
	Rank	37	28

$**p < .01$
$*p < .05$

NOTES TO APPENDIX

1. Gail Stuart, "How Professional Is Nursing?," *Images: The Journal of Nursing Scholarship* 13 (1981): 18–23.

2. Virginia Cleland, "The Professional Model," *American Journal of Nursing,* 75 (1975): 288–292.

3. Ada Jacox, "Collective Action: The Basis for Professionalism," *Supervisor Nurse,* Sept. 1980, pp. 22–32.

4. Margretta M. Styles, *On Nursing: Toward a New Endowment* (St. Louis, Mo.: C.V. Mosby, 1982).

5. Ibid.

6. Ibid., p. 8.

7. Ibid.

8. Ibid., pp. 74–76.

9. Lyman W. Porter, "Job Attitudes in Management," *Journal of Applied Psychology* 46 (1962): 375–384.

10. Yeager and Kline, "Professional Assn. Membership of Nurses: Factors Affecting Membership and the Decision to Join an Association," *Research in Nursing and Health,* 6 (1983): 48–52.

Part III

Chapter 5

The Nurse as a Colleague of the Physician

Joyce Patricia Brockhaus, R.N., M.S.N., Ph.D.
Anne T. Richardson, R.N., M.S.N.

INTRODUCTION

The subject of this chapter is the concept of collegiality between nurses and physicians. The literature contains many references to positive collaborative/collegial relationships between practicing nurses and doctors. Mauksch states that improvement of the present system of health delivery tops the list of reasons why solid relationships between nurses and physicians are beneficial: "Because nurses and physicians constitute the principal provider dyad of patient care delivery, it is reasonable to assume that the quality of their relationship is a determinant of the quality of patient care they deliver."[1] There are two important aspects of this statement: the quality of the nurse-physician relationship, and the quality of patient care resulting from that relationship.

Our examination of collegiality will include the historical development of interactions between the two professions. The problems and potential of colleague relationships between nursing and medicine will be treated, and recommendations will be offered for enhancing the development and maintenance of collaborative partnerships between the two professions.

WHY COLLEGIALITY?

In the 1960s, organized medicine and nursing began to state publicly that the discord growing between nurses and doctors needed to be settled. The hostility and lack of communication between the two professions was straining further a troubled health care system. The need for collaboration, realigned roles, and team effort was discussed at conferences and written about in publications. The impetus for collegiality between nursing and medicine has stemmed primarily from the nursing profession: it is nurses who desire a change in the relationship that exists between the two professions.

Collegiality implies a relationship that epitomizes collaborative working. It connotes equality, mutuality, rights, privileges, and power: qualities that enhance human productivity. An almost emotional component is found in Styles's discussion of collegiality: "A sacred vow; a solemn promise whereby we bind ourselves to those who share our cause, our convictions, our identity, our destiny."[2] The destiny, the enhanced human productivity, is the betterment of health care provided by nursing and medicine. It is the betterment of quality and quantity with the reduction of risk and cost to the individuals receiving health care services as well as to the individuals and institutions providing them. A state of productivity is the "what" collegiality provides.

However, "why" collegiality contributes to productivity is frequently subtle and complex. Styles reiterates that through collegiality "individual endeavor is potentiated, not pooled—respect then follows, with the acknowledgement and encouragement of the contribution that others make to our mutual task."[3] Collegiality can then be viewed not as a goal in and of itself but as a result of other goals: the goals of fostering oneself and one's profession as well as the goal of inherent enhancement of other professions when a mutual endeavor is involved. Hence, equality, mutuality, rights, privileges, and power are characteristics of one's profession and contribute to the overall outcome.

Even though medicine has become more and more dependent on other professions to be most effective, there is still a resistance to this change as is evident in Lee's study in which 22.3 percent of physicians questioned approval of collegial relationships between nursing and medicine.[4] Are the key words here "dependent on?" Is this the reason for not wanting collegiality? Do these words bring about a fear of loss of rights, privileges, and power of one's own profession? Indeed they could if they were meant to impose and dictate. However, if the words "dependent on" were used to mean "depend on," then they would reflect the core of collegiality as represented by the Latin root *collega*, meaning "one chosen to serve with another," choosing to work with others to accomplish more than one can accomplish on one's own.[5] For what possible reason would one not want collegiality?

WHAT IS A COLLEAGUE?

An attempt to define the term "colleague" reveals that the word carries connotations of both work and status.

The work or occupational component helps to distinguish collegiality from other types of relationships. Similarities in work type facilitate the usage of "colleague": people within the same profession refer to one another as colleagues. People of different professions who collaborate on a project might refer to each other as colleagues: a scientist and a physician working together on a research project or a biologist, anthropologist, and archeologist working together on a dig.

However, not all work situations connote occupation and are therefore not apt to use collegial terminology to denote relationship. For example, spouses do not generally refer to each other as colleagues in child rearing.

The second component is that of status. Often "colleague" is reserved for those who engage in work at a certain recognized prestigious level—a level denoted as "professional." Lawyers, physicians, dentists, educators, and politicians may refer to those within their respective professions as colleagues, and they may also give equal recognition to individuals in other professions if they deem that profession equal in status. Those individuals engaged in an occupation not generally recognized as professional refrain from using the terminology of colleague. For example, one would not expect to hear clerks at the supermarket or salespeople in department stores describe their coworkers as colleagues. Likewise, those engaged in sports would not use the term colleague unless practicing their skills at a professional level.

Since the concept of professional is key to the understanding of collegiality, the definition of professional needs to be considered. Larson states that there are certain criteria that must be met for a job to be a profession; specifically, that it must have: (1) a social market for its skills; (2) some exclusiveness for these skills; (3) an educational component; (4) some status gained for its members; and (5) some auto-regulation or governing organization.[6]

How do nursing and medicine measure up as professions according to these criteria? (See Chapter 8 for additional content.) Let's examine them with a view to the historical development of both professions.

Traditionally, the job of caring for the ill was given to the women in society. In earlier times, the ill and the handicapped were usually segregated and viewed as unproductive and worthless, yet cared for in some manner. There were no antibiotics, no tranquilizers, no suites of operating rooms; intensive care units and coronary care units were unheard of. It was a time in which physicians as well as nurses could do little more than provide palliative care for their patients. Because so little was known of how to remedy the illnesses and handicaps, the role of caring for the sick was restricted to doing what was possible to relieve pain and suffering.

While this early beginning to the profession of nursing might not have met Larson's criteria for a profession, there certainly was a social need, a market, for such a job. Although the skills might not have been exclusive, they were exhibited almost exclusively by women in most societies. Education in such skills was typically by word of mouth and trial and error. Status was low—in fact, caring for the sick was viewed as demeaning and unprestigious with very few rewards, valued surprisingly little by society.

The esteem associated with providing care for the ill came later with the investigation of ways to alter the course of certain illnesses and handicaps. While these experimental endeavors were looked on with skepticism in their early stages, the steady progress made in learning about the body and success in treating diseases eventually gained far more respect than did the business of simply "caring for" the sick. New discoveries, technologies, and opportunities in this century widened the gap between the two professions. Men were free to study and learn; women were not. Men went to the universities; women stayed at home. Medicine developed by leaps and bounds; nursing barely crept along.

The issue of marketing points out a real difference between the professions of nursing and medicine. Medicine required highly specialized services, while nursing was carried out by a group of individuals who were really just practicing skills that had been the realm of the general female population in earlier times. According to Larson, "If the technical base of an occupation consists of a vocabulary that sounds familiar to everyone, or if the base is scientific but so narrow that it can be learned as a set of rules by most people, then the occupation will have difficulty claiming a monopoly of skill or even a roughly exclusive jurisdiction."[7] Society expected members of the medical occupation to be experts because they possessed exclusive skills; it did not hold the same view of nursing.

The concept of marketing is unique for the nursing profession. What does nursing have to market? Nursing had always been linked with medicine as if to say that nursing could not exist without medicine. Recent controversy over independent nursing practitioners seems to reinforce the notion that nursing is an extension of medicine and therefore has no marketable skills of its own. Medicine seems to fear that nursing is becoming a separate profession, when often this is not the case. More often than not, nursing operates with some direct supervision or direction from the medical profession.

If the purpose of marketing is to acquire clients who pay for a service, the marketing of nursing falls short, since very little direct payment occurs between nurses and their "clients." The issue of valuing services, however, is an important aspect of the marketing of nursing. In a study by Blackwood, 90 percent of patients' reactions to hospitalization depended on the quality of care given by nurses.[8]

The second of Larson's criteria, the exclusiveness of skills, has brought the greatest controversy. Seldom have those in medicine questioned their job. Nursing, however, has not enjoyed such a clearly defined role. The question of what nursing is has been one that many in the profession have struggled with. Is nursing an extension of medicine—there to carry out only the limited aspects of "illness state" orientation? It is doubtful that many nurses would agree that they entered nursing solely to assist a physician in caring for patients. The recent American Nurses' Association social policy statement does an excellent job of addressing the issue of what nursing is.[9]

Can it be said that nursing provides skills and expertise not available through other services? The foundation of nursing is caring for people who are ill. There is a lot of "nurse" in all of us, for almost all human beings care for people who are ill at some time or another. While nurses cannot claim to provide a totally unique service, they do care for the sick at a level not possible by the average person. In this way, nursing is a unique and exclusive service.

The educational directions taken by these two occupations have also affected how each profession has come to be viewed. While nurses might have taught doctors how to comfort and care for the sick, that was not the true purpose of medicine. Medicine's goal was to alter and change, and physicians had to try new and different approaches to treating illness. As these changes were introduced, nurses had to learn how to incorporate them into their caring activities. The training of nurses in these new approaches was done by the physicians. Thus a strong foundation was laid for the directing of nurses by physicians. Knowledge, particularly the knowledge of medicine and healing, has always been valued by society and carries a tremendous amount of power. The licensing and awarding of degrees to physicians in recognition of their job preparation has traditionally set them apart from nursing.

Nowhere in our society can a physician obtain a license without extensive and exclusive postgraduate education. While there are a number of avenues available for the preparation of nurses, many of them do not require college, much less higher educational training. The educational preparation of nurses falls comparatively short of other professions, as evidenced by the fact that a low percentage of nurses have degrees of higher education. How does this affect the way in which the nursing profession is viewed? Larson, in examining the professions of teaching, law, and medicine, notes that the possession of advanced scientific education by colleges and universities, and by those who study there, makes the crucial difference between professional versus mere technical status.[10]

The reward system that developed around these two occupations has also been very different. The social status—prestige and power—that has been accorded those of the medical profession, as well as the financial rewards that accompany that status, have far surpassed those given to the nursing profession.

Finally, the self-regulation of the two occupations has differed from the beginning. Nurses do not enjoy the level of autonomy that physicians do. Frequently, hospitals have been controlled and regulated by physicians who kept a tight rein on the activities of nursing.

Using Larson's professional criteria as guideposts, it quickly becomes evident that nursing and medicine have not kept developmental pace. The differences in growth between the two professions have resulted in a gap in the relationship between them, a gap that threatens to grow wider unless the differences are explored and resolved.

The following section will examine in more detail the practical differences that have arisen in the roles of doctors and nurses, with a view to understanding, and thereby overcoming, the conflicts that interfere with the collegial interaction of nurse and physician.

FACTORS THAT HINDER COLLEGIALITY

Structuring of Work

Sheard discusses the ways in which nurses and physicians structure work differently. He states that,

> In performing the multiple tasks of a specific work role, individuals develop problem-solving methods, informal rules, and standard practices that help them organize and control their work. While the methods might not make sense to the outsider, to the practitioner they represent logical steps for accomplishing tasks.[11]

As long as those involved in different occupations share a common objective for an activity, they have a basis for cooperation and complementarity. However, when those same individuals approach a task from differing perspectives, their work concepts and methods show significant divergence. Members of each work group may expect the other to perceive the work in the same way they do. Because each group fails to appreciate the unique requirements of the other, they may place unreasonable demands on each other. Disruptive, disagreeable, and inappropriate work demands may be blocked by delaying tactics, subterfuge, or bargaining; thus, conflicts spiral and escalate.

The conflict that occurs between staff nurses and physicians in hospitals can be attributed to this clash of work roles and the resulting misunderstanding of respective methods and responsibilities. While their jobs are intended to complement each other, too often they work at crossed purposes. Some of the sources of these differences may be the following:

- sense of time
- sense of resources
- scope of practice
- work assignment
- reward system
- education
- sexual stereotypes[12]

These are areas that affect the practical, daily activities and interactions of nurses and physicians. As such, they offer the greatest potential for conflict and the best opportunity for cooperation. Let's analyze each detail to see how these divergent perspectives have evolved and how they might be brought together to enhance the collegial relationship.

Sense of Time

In their work, physicians have a sense of time marked not by the hour but by the course of illness or disease. Unexpected episodes in the course of illness serve as landmarks by which the physician measures the patient's progress toward recovery, invalidism, or death.

Physicians measure time in units, such as the number of days since surgery, length of a course of chemotherapy, and number of hours until a drug takes effect. The unit of time expands or contracts to meet the problem at hand and can be neither strictly scheduled nor easily measured.

Nurses, unlike physicians, have an hourly, strictly scheduled sense of time. Of necessity, their day is organized around a rigid schedule of tasks, their time ordered in blocks. In each block, a group of homogeneous tasks is performed, according to a daily worksheet. As the tasks are performed, they are crossed off the list until all the work is done.

Since physicians do not think in terms of a strictly organized eight-hour day, they may interpret the disruptions that arise from work schedules as nursing error. Without understanding these differences and why they exist, the two groups tend to react to each other out of ignorance and insensitivity.

Sense of Resources

Physicians have an "abundance" view of hospital resources. They write requests in the patient's chart with little awareness of the time and effort required to carry them out. In the past, the hospital offered physicians a nearly limitless pool of resources. As a result, many unnecessary tests or treatments were ordered, and nurses were prohibited by training and hospital policy from blocking physicians' excessive requests. Fortunately, economic necessity is forcing a change in the attitudes of physicians toward resources, as hospitals implement stricter policies that limit tests and treatment. Because physicians have always written requests easily, they have had a distorted sense of the ease with which the tasks may be carried out. They have rarely been involved as nurses have been in the difficulties of obtaining supplies and scheduling patients.

The fear of legal suits has also been a factor in the proliferation of tests and unnecessary diagnostic measures. In addition, new tests and treatments carried out as a part of physician training have resulted in excessive and unnecessary work.

Nurses, on the other hand, have always had a view that hospital resources are limited and difficult to obtain. They have developed this parsimonious attitude for two reasons. First, nurses have often met great resistance from hospital supply and information departments, particularly when carrying out unusual or untimely requests. It has often been extremely difficult to accomplish physicians' requests in accordance with hospital protocol. Serving as the bridge between written and executed orders, the nurse struggles to harmonize the physician's request with the hospital's intransigence.

Because of their heavy workload, nurses object when asked by physicians to carry out unnecessary or repetitive procedures. Nurses may attempt to reduce their workload by requesting that physicians discontinue such procedures. Physicians may interpret these requests as challenges to their judgment or as indifference or neglect on the part of the nurse and become impatient because they do not comprehend the nurse's rationale. Similarly, a nurse may act hastily to remove an IV or stop an antibiotic without appreciating the physician's caution and concern. Because nurses and physicians view these tasks from such different perspectives, conflict is created.

Scope of Practice

Physicians use a global or broad scope of practice. Diagnosis and treatment require a holistic approach to the diseased body, and medical authority demands that the physician be responsible for all patient-related problems, no matter how small. Thus, physicians organize all pertinent data around the individual patient.

As they make daily rounds, physicians discuss each patient until they arrive at the diagnosis and plan of treatment. It would be absurd for physicians to discuss all the x-rays taken that day or all the blood work, since all cases do not apply to the care of each individual patient.

By contrast, nurses who practice team nursing must broaden their scope of practice. They focus less on the patient's overall problems and progress and more on the completion of scheduled tasks. Because of the way in which their work is scheduled, nurses typically organize their work so that they take all the blood pressures, then all the temperatures and daily weights, after which they serve all the trays, set up all the baths, and so forth. Performing tasks in this way can result in losing an integrated sense of the relationship between task and patient. This structure of the nurses' workload arose as a result of the shortage of nurses and reflects the organizational policies and constraints experienced by the nursing profession.

Problems arise as well when a physician criticizes a nurse for failing to report an important symptom. What the physician usually does not realize is that a great number of nonmedical tasks require the nurse's time, from clerking to moving furniture to enforcing hospital rules, and the nurse may not have had the time to notice a change in a patient's symptoms.

Work Assignment

Physicians work with patients on a case-by-case basis. Usually, physicians have begun their association with a patient before hospitalization, and they maintain that relationship until and even after the patient's problem has been resolved. Except for a few specialists, physicians maintain responsibility for their patients, even when they are transferred to other nursing units within the hospital. A healthy patient-physician relationship requires the continuity provided by case assignment.

In contrast, nurses are usually assigned to the patient geographically by room number. Nurses' assignments vary daily, placing them in contact with many different patients. This practice of assigning nurses to rooms rather than to patients prevents nurses from developing ongoing relationships with patients.

Reward System

Physicians are paid a salary or fee for service, not an hourly wage. Physicians do not think in terms of dollars per hour, or time-and-a-half for working late. Physicians' rewards for service are consistent with their global view of work, their enduring relationship with the patient, and their assignment by case.

Nurses are paid an hourly wage. This salary structure reinforces the scarcity view of resources and the short-term, strictly scheduled sense of time that has come to be characteristic of the nursing profession. Use of an hourly wage reinforces the short-term scope of their work and erodes the dedication to service and sense of professionalism with which most nurses begin their career.

The large differences in salaries and wages between physicians and nurses further contribute to the discord between the two groups.

The Educational Gap

Historically, nurses and physicians have not studied together, nor have their courses of study supplied either group with information about the contribution of the other to health care. Christman recognized the difference in educational preparation and its contribution to the fact that physicians and nurses value different aspects of health care. Even as more and more nurses receive graduate training, differences in emphasis in training continue to be a source of communication and care difficulties. The gap in education, and the focus of training, results in vast differences in perceptions of each other and of the health care field. Consequently, nurse and physician may work side by side throughout their professional lives without really understanding the other's point of view.[13]

Sexual Stereotypes

Since even in these changing times the majority of physicians are men and the majority of nurses are women, the nurse-physician relationship has followed the cultural pattern of male dominance and female subservience. The nurse has been conditioned to accept this relationship even to the point that she may address the physician as "doctor" while it is perfectly acceptable for the physician to refer to the nurse by her first name.

The physician views the physician-patient relationship as primary; all other care, including that given by nurses, is secondary. Felch noted that while some physicians recognize the emerging role of the nurse, many are threatened by it and therefore oppose it. He further stated that in order to resolve the conflict, role definitions for both the physician and the nurse are essential.[14] The AMA Council on Medical Education reported in 1977 that a major area of friction would be eliminated if physicians were to recognize the nurses as independent health care professionals practicing nursing under license and legally accountable to the consumer. In this way, nurses and physicians might develop a constructive and interdependent role.

SUMMARY OF PROBLEMS

It is evident that conflict has long plagued staff nurses and physicians in their working relationships. While they may present an image of harmony and cooperation to the public, there are often concealed misunderstandings, resentment, and anger. Conflict occurs because the work of nurses and physicians is structured in radically different ways, and although they work side by side, they tend to misunderstand one another's methods and motivations. This combination of differing approaches and lack of knowledge weakens the complementary nature of their respective roles and produces frustration and conflict.

Must there be conflict? Are there ways in which conflict can be reduced and, in fact, cooperative relationships be created? There are, and suggestions for finding those ways follow.

RECOMMENDATIONS TO ENHANCE COLLEGIALITY

Physicians are concerned primarily with the identification of disease and strategies for treatment and cure. Nurses, on the other hand, are concerned primarily with nurturing, caring, helping to cope, comforting, counseling, and providing life-supporting activities. The two professions, however, have mutual and overlapping concerns and responsibilities for patients.

Nurses and physicians work best as colleagues when there is:

- mutual agreement on a goal,
- equality in status and personal interactions,
- a shared base of scientific and professional knowledge,
- respect for complementary diversity in skills, expertise, and practice,
- mutual trust and respect for each other's competence, and
- open and effective communication.

Cooperative Patient Care

Through nursing organizations inside and outside of the hospital, nurses should encourage and work for primary nursing in contrast to team nursing or functional nursing models. In this way, they would have first-hand experience with the patients and could describe conditions to the physicians more accurately. Moreover, this global approach to patient care is closer to that of physicians and helps foster a common viewpoint. It allows both professionals to develop mutual goals in the delivery of patient care. Nurses would have a similar "investment" in the development of treatment goals, delivery of patient care, and evaluation of treatment success.

Primary nursing also gives nurses the visibility they need to be involved in care decisions: nurse and physician work together to establish priorities and goals, identify and evaluate problems, and recognize each other's individual competencies, methods, and personalities. A patient system that integrates the observations, judgments, and actions of nurses and physicians will reflect and contribute to collaborative practice and provide a method of formalizing nurse-physician communication in the care of patients.

In implementing this step, separate nurses' and doctors' progress notes should be eliminated. Instead, patient progress notes, and all written contributions to patient care, would share the same pages. Nurses often complain that doctors do not read nurses' notes, but in many cases, nurses do not read doctors' notes. Writing in the same place promotes each party's awareness of the other's contributions.

Team conferences discussing patient progress should be encouraged by both doctors and nurses whenever possible. The staff nurses can participate in daily rounds with the physician, communicating about treatment goals and contributing suggestions and information on a patient's progress.

A joint practice committee that gives equal representation to practicing nurses and physicians and that is supported by the hospital administration can monitor nurse-physician relationships and recommend appropriate actions supporting joint practice.

Nurses and doctors should share responsibility in making decisions about the needs and problems of patients. Contributions from nurses about the care required should be based on nursing theory and contributions from physicians on medical theory. Both, however, share common scientific bases and have equal value.

Education

Physicians cannot be expected to accept the decisions of nurses if they have no confidence in nurses' knowledge, skills, or judgment. It is the nurse's responsibility to keep abreast of current practices, as well as the hospital management's job to be sure that the nursing staff has the clinical preparation necessary to meet new standards of performance. Giving nurses more responsibility without adequate training is an invitation to further discord.

To exercise their professional clinical skills to the fullest, nurses must be encouraged to make individual clinical nursing decisions, with both medical and nursing consultation available on request. These decisions must be within the scope of nursing practice as defined within the hospital. Clinical competence is built in various ways: by writing specific performance standards; aggressive inservice education; and utilization of highly trained clinical nurse specialists to serve as role models and to provide on-the-job education. Clinical competence leads to clinical credibility. Too often, nurses err by demanding acceptance from physicians before demonstrating their competence.

Medical and nursing schools should provide collaborative courses that clearly explain nursing and medical roles. This type of interaction fosters and promotes mutual respect and provides an opportunity for nursing and medical students to develop informal as well as professional relationships.

The benefit of this arrangement is the exposure each discipline has to the other during the formative educational years and throughout professional training. Interdisciplinary educational efforts to date have been few and simplistic. Medical and nursing students who learn together should gain an understanding of and respect for each other's professional role that will remain with them and create a positive force for collaboration throughout their careers. Joint publication, shared research activities, and program development are prime examples of collaborative practices.

There is a trend toward decreasing the years required for obtaining the medical degree and increasing the years and scope of education for nurses at the preparatory level. Increasing numbers of nurses are obtaining advanced degrees in nursing, which prepare them for leadership in clinical practice, teaching, management, research, and consultation. While this trend will help close the educational gap, it will not remedy the situation altogether. The resolution of the education-credentials problem lies in recognizing, accepting, and rewarding the individual for competence, not just for the years spent in formal academic preparation.

Communication

In hospitals, communication problems between physicians and nurses often are allowed to continue without resolution, leading to an undercurrent of defensiveness that hampers effective patient care. It is the responsibility of hospital management to create a problem-solving structure to resolve work problems as swiftly and effectively as possible. When a nurse has difficulty with a physician, or a physician with a nurse, the structure for recourse for such problems would be clearly defined and promptly implemented. A person within the hospital system who is trained to assist with the constructive resolution of conflicts is of value. Inservice education programs on communication skills and problem solving can be beneficial as well.

Only by the utilization of effective communication skills and clearly defined problem-solving structures can we begin to move toward problem resolution and better working relationships.

Societal Issues

Nursing professionals must assert themselves by demonstrating their competence and by replacing their traditional role of submission to one of equality with men, irrespective of the hierarchical structures in their work situations.

A further challenge is presented by the lower prestige and pay accorded nurses. Until society recognizes the worth of the services rendered by nurses as fully as it recognizes and accepts the worth of the services rendered by physicians, this will remain a problem. Nurses must work actively within hospital communities and professional associations for recognition of their valuable contributions.

Nurses' involvement in the community as lobbyists, educators, researchers, board members, consultants, health care experts, and media spokespersons affords them the opportunity for this recognition.

SUMMARY

Our review of the development of the nurse-physician relationship has revealed some of the reasons why that relationship has fallen far short of its ideal.

The elimination of the barriers to constructive nurse-physician relationships will take a good deal of time and effort, but it is not an impossible task. The section on recommendations offers some practical first steps. The seeds of change have been planted: it is up to us to see that they are nurtured and encouraged to grow.

NOTES

1. Ingeborg G. Mauksch, "Nurse-Physician Collaboration: A Changing Relationship," *Journal of Nursing Administration,* June 1981, p. 35.

2. Margretta M. Styles, *On Nursing: Toward a New Endowment* (St. Louis, Mo.; C. V. Mosby Co., 1982), p. 143.

3. Ibid.

4. Anthony A. Lee, "How Nurses Rate with M.D.'s: Still the Handmaiden." *RN,* July 1979, p. 22.

5. *The Grolier International Dictionary* (Danbury, CT: Grolier Incorporated, 1980).

6. Magali Sarfatti Larson, *The Rise of Professionalism: A Sociological Analysis* (Los Angeles: University of California Press, 1977), p. 96.

7. Ibid., p. 121.

8. Sarah A. Blackwood, "At This Hospital, 'The Captain of the Ship' is Dead," *RN,* March 1979, p. 85.

9. American Nurses' Association, *Nursing—A Social Policy Statement* (Kansas City, Mo.: American Nurses' Association, 1980), pp. 9–20.

10. Magali Sarfatti Larson, *The Rise of Professionalism: A Sociological Analysis* (Los Angeles: University of California Press, 1977), p. 125.

11. Timothy Sheard, "The Structure of Conflict in Nurse-Physician Relations," *Supervisor Nurse*, August 11, 1980, p. 14.

12. Ibid.

13. Luther Christman, "Nurse-Physician Communication in the Hospital," *Journal of the American Medical Association,* November 1965, p. 539.

14. W. C. Felch, "Physician-Nurse Relationships," *Hospital Medical Staff,* July 1976, p. 6.

SUGGESTED READINGS

Altschul, A. "With All Due Respect . . . Interprofessional Relations." *Nursing Mirror* 157, no. 2 (July 13, 1983): 20.

American Nurses' Association. *Nursing—A Social Policy Statement.* Kansas City, Mo.: ANA, 1980.

Blackwood, Sarah A. "At This Hospital 'The Captain of the Ship' is Dead," *RN*, March 1979, p. 77–94.

Chaska, Norma L., ed. *The Nursing Profession: Views Through the Mist.* New York: McGraw-Hill Book Co., 1978.

Chaska, Norma L. *The Nursing Profession: A Time to Speak.* New York: McGraw-Hill Book Co., 1983.

Devereux, Pamela M. "Essential Elements of Nurse-Physician Collaboration." *Journal of Nursing Administration* 5 (May 11, 1981): 19–23.

Devereux, Pamela M. "Nurse/Physician Collaboration: Nursing Practice Considerations." *Journal of Nursing Administration,* September 1981, pp. 37–39.

DeYoung, Carol; Tower, Margene; and Glittenburg, Jody. *Out of Uniform and into Trouble, Again: The Nurse's Role in Community Mental Health Centers and Other Places.* Thorofare, N.J.: Slack, Inc., 1971, pp. 22–34.

"Doctors, Nurses Must Discuss Differences, Work Together." *Hospitals* 52, no. 24 (December 16, 1978): 17–18.

Dopson, L. "Lines of Communication." *Nursing Times* 75, no. 14 (April 5, 1979): 567.

Duespohl, T.A. *Nursing in Transition.* Rockville, Md.: Aspen Systems Corp., 1983.

Erde, E. L. "Notions of Teams and Team Talk in Health Care: Implications for Responsibilities." *Law-Med-Health-Care* 9, no. 5 (October 1981): 26–28.

Floyd, Gloria Jo, and Smith, Billy Don. "Job Enrichment." *Nursing Management* 14, no. 5 (May 1983): 22.

Friedman, F. B. "A Nurse's Guide to the Care and Handling of MDs." *RN* 45, no. 3 (March 1982): 39–43, 118–120.

Furnham, A.; Pendleton, D.; and Manicom, C. "The Perception of Different Occupations Within the Medical Profession." *Soc-Sci-Med (E),* November 1981, pp. 289–300.

Gillies, Dee Ann. *Nursing Management: A Systems Approach.* Philadelphia: Saunders, 1982, pp. 150–159.

Giovinco, G. "Interpersonal/Professional Relationship: Some Critical Issues Involving the Nurse, the Physician and the Patient." *Journal of Nursing Ethics* 1, no. 1 (Fall 1978): 13–16.

Glen, S. "Stop Pandering to Doctors." *Nursing Mirror* 154, no. 25 (June 23, 1982): 48–49.

Grubb, L. L. "Nurse-Physician Collaboration." *Supervisor Nurse* 10, no. 3 (March 1979): 16–21.

Hirata, I. Jr. "Togetherness—The Health Care Team." *J-Am-Coll-Health Assoc.* 29, no. 1 (August 1980): 5–6.

Hofling, Charles K. et al. "An Experimental Study in Nurse-Physician Relationships." *The Journal of Mental and Nervous Disease* 143, no. 2: 171–180.

Johnston, P. F. "Improving the Nurse-Physician Relationship." *Journal of Nursing Administration* 13, no. 3 (March 1983): 19–20.

Lang, D. A. and Goertzen, I. "Doctors vs Nurses: Is Anybody Winning?" *Nurs-Careers* 2, no. 4 (September–October 1981): 16–17.

Larson, Magali Sarfatti. *The Rise of Professionalism—A Sociological Analysis.* Los Angeles: University of California Press, 1977.

Lee, A. A. "How Nurses Rate with MDs: Still the Handmaiden." *RN* 42, no. 7 (July 1979): 20–30.

Lynch, B. L. "Team Building: Will it Work in Health Care?" *Journal of Allied Health* 10, no. 4 (November 1981): 240–247.

Marriner, Ann. *The Nursing Process: A Scientific Approach to Nursing Care.* St. Louis, Mo.: C. V. Mosby Co., 1975.

Martin, J. C. "Hospital Problems Need Interprofessional Approach." *Dimens-Health-Serv.* 56, no. 8 (August 1979): 8–9.

Mauksch, Ingeborg, G., and Miller, Michael H. *Implementing Change in Nursing.* St. Louis, Mo.: C. V. Mosby Co., 1981, pp. 73–86.

Mauksch, Ingeborg G. "Nurse-Physician Collaboration: A Changing Relationship." *Journal of Nursing Administration* 11, no. 6 (June 1981): 35–38.

McGuire, M. A. "Nurse-Physician Interactions: Silence Isn't Golden." *Supervisor Nurse* 11, no. 3 (March 11, 1980): 36–39.

Morgan, A. P., and McCann, J. M. "Nurse-Physician Relationships: The Ongoing Conflict." *Nursing Administration Quarterly* 7, no. 4 (Summer 1983): 1–7.

Murphy, L. M. "War Lords One, Nurses Zero." *RN* 41, no. 10 (October 1978): 45–46.

Pawsat, E. H. "The New Horizon Nurse and the Physician: A Need for Guidelines." *Wis-Med-J* 80, no. 11 (November 1981): 15–17.

Phillips, J. R. "Health Care Provider Relationships a Matter of Reciprocity." *Nursing Outlook* 27, no. 11 (November 1979): 738–741.

Pluckhan, Margaret L. "Professional Territoriality: A Problem Affecting the Delivery of Health Care." *Nursing Forum* 11, no. 3 (1972): 300–310.

Ride, T. "Do We Understand the Process?" *Nursing Mirror* 157, no. 7 (August 17, 1983): 12–13.

Ritter, H. A. "Nurse-Physician Collaboration." *Conn-Med* 45, no. 1 (January 1981): 23–25.

Rodgers, J. A. "Toward Professional Adulthood." *Nursing Outlook* 29, no. 8 (August 1981): 478–481.

Schreckenberger, Paul C. "Playing for the Health Team." *J.A.M.A.* 213, no. 2 (July 30, 1970): 279–281.

Schwartzbaum, A.; McGrath, J. H.; and Byrd, L. H. Jr. "Doctor, Brush Up Your Manners!" *RN* 46, no. 5 (May 1983): 64–65.

Sheard, T. "The Structure of Conflict in Nurse-Physician Relations." *Supervisor Nurse* 11, no. 8 (August 1980): 14–18.

Shumaker, D., and Goss, V. "Toward Collaboration: One Small Step." *Nurs-Health-Care* 1, no. 4 (November 1980): 183–185.

Singleton, A. F. "Physician-Nurse Perceptions of Styles of Power Usage." *Social-Sci-Med (E)* 15, no. 3 (August 1981): 231–237.

Sovik, W. E. "Physician-Nurse Relationship From the Physician Viewpoint." *Ohio-State-Med-J* 76, no. 1 (January 1980): 37–38.

Stanley, I. "Accountability in Nursing. Where do We Stand with Doctors?" *Nurs-Times* 79, no. 38 (September 21–27, 1983): 46–48.

Stein, Leonard I. "The Doctor-Nurse Game." *Archives of General Psychiatry* 16 (June 1967): 699–703.

Styles, Margretta M. *On Nursing: Toward a New Endowment.* St. Louis, Mo.: C. V. Mosby Co., pp. 142–150.

Styles, Margretta M. "Reflections on Collaboration and Unification." *Image: The Journal of Nursing Scholarship* 16, no. 1 (Winter 1984): 21–23.

Sumner, E. "Time to Overturn 'Doctor's Law'." *Nursing Times* 77, no. 43 (October 28–November 3, 1981): 1874.

Torrez, Sister Mary Rachel. "Systems Approach to Staffing." *Nursing Management* 14, no. 5 (May 1983): 54.

Trinosky, P. "Nurse-Doctor Dissension Still Thrives." *Supervisor Nurse* 10, no. 4 (April 1979): 40–43.

Wilson, J. "Ethics and the Physician-Nurse Relationship." *Can-Med-Assoc.-J.* 129, no. 3 (August 1, 1983): 290–293.

Winker, Cynthia K., and Lee, Nancy C. "Developing a Joint Practice Team." *Dimensions of Critical Care Nursing* 1, no. 6 (November/December 1982): 360–363.

Wise, Harold; Rubin, Irwin; and Beckard, Richard. "Making Health Teams Work." *American Journal of Diseases in Children* 127 (April 1974): 537–542.

Chapter 6

Nursing Interfacing with Nursing

Audrey Kalafatich, R.N., Ed.D., F.A.A.N.
Robin Moushey, R.N., M.S.N.

INTRODUCTION

This chapter addresses the issues inherent in nurses collaborating with each other. The first section considers collaboration in nursing practice, including nursing administration. The second section deals with collaboration among practice, nursing education, and nursing research.

Collaboration appears to be the word of the hour. Various styles of collaboration are related in reviewing current literature, including chapters in this book. The literature often describes physician-nurse collaboration, which focuses on developing reciprocity between these professions and other health care professionals. However, the literature concerning the collaborative practice that exists or should exist within nursing is not that abundant. Two assumptions can be made: (1) this process is already at full momentum, or (2) it is time to scrutinize the ways in which nurses deal with other nurses.

To describe nursing interfacing with nursing, the word "collaboration" needs to be explored. Styles has stated that "collaboration is working together—processes, purposes and pitfalls notwithstanding."[1] It sounds simple, but the complexity of the process increases with implementation.

The increased utilization of the collaborative process coincides with the impact of the primary nursing system. According to Carper, Orem has said that the art of nursing is "expressed by the individual nurse through her creativity and style in designing and providing nursing that is effective and satisfying."[2] Collaboration needs to be incorporated into that statement. Nursing has diversified into a variety of roles committed to the united goal of quality of patient care. None of these roles can function effectively without the utilization of the other's expertise. That is where collaboration is an integral part of the health care system. When one, two, or three nurses decide that patients and their families require more interventions for adaptation on the health-illness continuum than one nurse can offer, then collaboration takes place.

NURSING INTERFACING WITH NURSING IN INSTITUTIONAL PRACTICE

Nursing Practice

The social policy statement issued by the American Nurses' Association describes collaboration as "true partnership, power on both sides is valued by both, the recognition and acceptance of separate and combined spheres of activity and responsibility, mutual safeguarding of the legitimate interest of each party, and a commonality of goals that is recognized by both parties."[3] How is this description manifested in the clinical setting? Commonality of goals is fairly easy to accomplish: most nurses, regardless of roles, strive for similar outcomes of quality patient care. One cannot speak as easily of partnership and power. Therein lies the complexity of nurse-nurse collaboration. Through various activities, nurses may see common goals but they may not perceive implementing these goals through the same interventions. How does one intertwine role diversity and power in the process of collaboration in the clinical setting?

The social policy statement alludes to the differences in nursing roles. "Instead of homogeneity (a nurse is a nurse is a nurse), there is heterogeneity of clinical interests and levels of competence within nursing."[4] Surely there are differences in nursing activity, but the essence of nursing should be the core of every role. As the social policy states, variances within the clinical setting stem from differences in educational background, clinical experience, and competence. These variances are evident in clinical settings where there are primary nurses, clinical nurse specialists, and student nurses caring for the clients and their families. However different their competency levels may be, each has to value the other as an integral part of the caring process or else the collaborative modality will be lost. Nurses bring a part of themselves, a part of their values, and a part of their expertise in order to accomplish common goals.

The discussion of role and influence brings up the question of the use of power in the collaborative process. The power that plays a part in the collaborative process has to be unified on all sides. Each individual is contributing to the whole to create a power that can be shared. It should be "ongoing, interactive and dynamic."[5]

French and Raven speak to the five basics of power: (1) reward, (2) coercive, (3) expert, (4) reverent, and (5) legitimate.[6] What basics of power are inherent in the clinical setting? (The nursing administration role is discussed further in the chapter, so emphasis here is on the clinical component.) Reward power obviously rewards for compliance to another's plan. Coercive power is power that is highly persuasive. Unfortunately, it may bear a negative connotation. Expert power alludes to influence based on a superior knowledge base. Reverent power describes power based on the influence of the individual's characteristics on the clinical situation. Legitimate power lies within the position held or is inherent in a given role.

When nurses have varying roles, power should be utilized as a shared process. Power that can be utilized readily in the collaborative process would be reward, expert, and reverent power. Each nurse working in collaboration with another can reward that person, can share his or her expertise, and can influence his or her communication, style, and personality. This can be accomplished easily without confusion or conflict in roles if there is an open and trusting communication pattern.

Communication is the start of collaboration. Styles describes the hierarchy of elements of collaboration in terms of people as the baseline, with other elements being purposes, principles, and then structure.[7] Consultation begins at the first element of hierarchy, which involves those nurses in the clinical setting. Styles discusses the stages necessary to develop a unified structure. She states that it begins with a nonrelationship, which progresses to communication, consultation, consent, unified policy, and, the last step, unified structure.[8]

"Communication" is the key word in this process. Literature relates much information on the function of various clinical roles in the consulting process. However, the consultant is powerless unless integrated into the system by a consultee. That consultee has to visualize the consultant as an asset in reaching nursing goals. This role should be supportive and complementary and not a sign that the consultee is unable to accomplish the task at hand.

The nurse can adapt to concerns in the clinical setting by consulting and collaborating with others. Roy speaks of adaptations and stimuli. Stimuli have been described as focal, or those immediately confronting the person; contextual, or all other stimuli present; and residual, or the beliefs, attitudes, and experience of the individual.[9] The consultation/collaborative process links closely with this theory. Staff nurses assess what is immediately confronting them in the clinical situation (focal stimuli). Nurses have to see how this immediate client concern affects the rest of the clinical setting (contextual stimuli). The overall picture is then viewed through the eyes of the nurses' own beliefs, attitudes, and experiences (residual stimuli). This is the process whereby a consultant is summoned.

The people who request a consultant can be as varied as the consultants themselves. Krakowski describes six types of consultees.[10] The eager consultees are so filled with anxiety and possible failure that they seek help in any form. Unfortunately, their anxiety may cloud the assessment of the situation. A reciprocal consultation is termed "one-for-one." Consultation is done rather as a courtesy, and the party asking may not be truly interested in what the consultant has to say. The forgetful consultee may feel obliged to ask for the consult, but does little follow-up with the advice. The apologetic consultee may lead the client to believe that the consultation may be a bother, and no heed has to be paid to the consultant's assessment. The expert consultees have all the answers. They only consider consultation to validate their own assessment or intervention. If the consultants disagree, the consultees may quickly agree to avoid confrontation or simply disregard the advice. If the consultants do disagree, they are seldom asked for further advice.

As the previous discussion easily predicts, the act of calling on a consultant does not necessarily result in a true consultation or collaborative practice. "Consultation requires mutual trust and respect; power or support is acquired by creating a need, filling a gap and finally achieving credibility."[11] This trust and mutual respect requires an openness for the utilization of all aspects of nursing roles and functions. Persons need to be open to role versatility as well as to one another. "Openness includes availability in terms of time, receptiveness, and responsiveness to staff opinions and feelings and demonstrations of humaneness."[12]

Consultation in no way automatically breeds consent. The stage from consultation to consent is also a complex one when dealing with situations involving change. Nursing and change are almost synonymous. However, nursing staff are notorious for resisting change in any shape or form. Therefore it takes effort to change consult to consent in nursing decisions.

Let's look at change in the clinical setting. The process from consulting to consenting may connotate change for one or both parties involved in the collaborative process. It can also involve the client who could be shifting position on the health-illness continuum. Kasch has stated that the goal of nursing is to maximize adaptation.[13] In order for collaboration to become a thriving process, some adaptation has to be promoted for all parties involved. Nurses help clients to adapt, and nurses should also help other nurses to adapt.

What are the factors that help the consultee adapt to the changes that may occur as a result of the collaborative process? Adapting conserves energy.[14] Resistance usually calls for more hard work. "Resistance is a behavior which attempts to protect the person from the effects of real or imagined change."[15] Resistance to change can be avoided, and Miller has stated various ways this can be done:

- treating people as individuals,
- involving those affected in planning,
- providing accurate and complete information,
- giving time to air objections,
- taking group norms or behavior into account,
- making only essential changes,
- utilizing problem-solving techniques,
- gaining support of top officials,
- providing an avenue for feedback, and
- being open to feelings about revision of the plan.[16]

Openness and trust are evident when one treats individuals with respect. Mutual trust is gained when each party values the information obtained through the collaborative process. The information shared in the collaboration process has to be involved in a continual feedback situation. Consultants who perform one-time assessments miss their mark when no follow-up or evaluation is instituted by the consultee or consultant. By involving people in a decision-making process, their involvement and commitment will greatly increase.

Miller makes an astute statement clarifying that only essential changes should be made. Change for change's sake only serves to disturb the need for some stabilization in the clinical setting. By making only essential changes, group norms and behaviors are taken into account. Consultants have to be keenly aware of the climate of the clinical setting at the time that they are making assessments and planning for intervention. What worked with the last client last week may not be appropriate for the present setting. By using the problem-solving process, feelings and concerns can be discussed openly prior to any intervention being planned. Through this same process, feedback from outcomes can be processed, and evaluation can be initiated.

Let us look at what is happening in reality in the clinical setting. How well are we collaborating with our variety of roles and role functions? In discussing nursing interacting with nursing, the subject of the clients and their families has not been addressed directly. It needs to be stated that the collaborative process is not complete without input from client and family. However, the subject of clients and families will be fully addressed in another chapter, and the assumption should be made that they are continually involved with nursing interfacing with nursing.

This chapter has related what the "experts" believe about collaborative practice. What thoughts interplay in the staff nurse's mind? The nurses are the force that will make or break a collaborative entity. A small survey was developed to elicit ideas from the staff nurses in describing collaboration. This form is shown in Exhibit 6-1.

On surveying staff nurses, one derives the following definitions of collaboration: "Combining resources to reach a common goal. A combination of people working together with different information to plan the care of a patient." This statement coincides with what the experts state.

Other nurses describe the collaborative process as working together for an ultimate goal. They stated the need to incorporate different services, departments, physicians, and nurses in the collaborative process. Key phrases in their descriptions were "sharing," "working together," and "helping." Combining efforts for the ultimate goal of improved patient care outcomes was the evident theme.

Exhibit 6-1

Please fill out briefly.　Name:
　　　　　　　　　　　Unit:
1. What does collaboration mean to you?
2. With whom do you collaborate? (1 = most often used, 2 = next utilized,
　3 = sometimes utilized, 4 = seldom utilized, 5 = never utilized)

　　＿＿＿＿＿ Associate Nurse/Staff Nurse
　　＿＿＿＿＿ Clinical Nurse Specialist
　　＿＿＿＿＿ Clinical Nurse
　　＿＿＿＿＿ Clinical Advisor
　　＿＿＿＿＿ Patient Care Manager

How do you collaborate?　　　　　　　　　　　Yes　No　Sometimes

Actual consultation

Informal discussions

Care planning (documentation)

Core group—conference

One staff nurse gave a somewhat different explanation. "It means compromising even though you may not really want to. Individuals uniting their efforts to complete a task." This describes the concerns that the consultee may experience when contacting a consultant. Collaboration may evoke the need to change an approach in the clinical setting, and this change often evokes friendly resistance within the collaborative process. These sentiments also coincide with the earlier discussion on some of the pitfalls of collaboration and change.

In relating with whom they collaborate in the clinical setting, nurses gave other staff nurses the highest rating for consultation. In Styles's model of the elements of collaboration, her first steps in the staircase are people who are the staff nurses in the situation. Minute to minute, day to day, staff nurses collaborate with their peers.

Peers may be experienced nurses or young graduates. The experienced nurse has a certain amount of influence in the clinical setting. Varricchio describes influence as the "provision of relevant information by one person to another who takes that information into account when arriving at a decision."[17] This influence has the potential to evolve into power. Any individual who has worked in a nursing unit is aware of those individuals, regardless of rank, who can yield power within the system. Power can be seen as an influence to ways of getting results.[18] Nurses were often educated in an environment that dictated parental influence through the utilization of dorm mothers and clinical instructors who allowed little autonomy from their students. This environment persisted when the young student graduated and confronted a nursing unit flooded with supervisors, head nurses, assistant head nurses, team leaders, and so on. It is no wonder that collaboration was not spoken of widely in those clinical situations. How can one collaborate when one is terrified of asking a question?

However, things changed. Power became decentralized through the innovative actions of various nursing managers. These actions probably occurred from the influence of nurses who were changing themselves: no longer were nurses handmaidens to others. Social awareness of the role of women, as well as altering practices in nursing education, influenced the role of new staff nurses. Nurses became more challenged and motivated with their evolving role, yet they still possessed some uncertainties. Risk-taking was not foreign to these new nurses. Nurses were willing to toss their plans of intervention of nursing care into the ring of ideas of other health care professionals. This meant that they were capable of not being overwhelmed by the influence of the more experienced nurses. They could seek out information openly and also utilize their assessment skills to determine if the knowledge shared would contribute to the given situation. The experienced nurse would still have influence and utilize power in the reward, reverent, and expertise domains. The loss of power sould be in the coercive domain. Nursing roles that had influence bordering on power have been described as information-givers. As decentralization continues in the practice setting, nurses are viewed as having equal and mutual power. Influences can be a changing pattern depending on each clinical situation and those individuals involved in the collaboration process.

Credibility accompanies a sharing of skills, knowledge, attitudes, and beliefs. Sharing can be accomplished only through involvement in the clinical setting. This availability is inherent in some roles. The clinical advisor, who functions as an assistant head nurse, was noted by the staff nurses to be second in their line of involvement in the process of collaboration. Clinical advisors tend to be available to their staff in planning day-to-day patient care interventions. They are utilized because they are there. "Being there" is essential to role utilization in the collaborative practice. Nurses cannot collaborate with other nurses who are not available and skilled in clinical practice. The skill of an experienced nurse evokes trust in others.

After mutual trust is reached in the collaborative setting, autonomy can be achieved. "Professional autonomy can be defined as both independent and interdependent practice related decision making based on a complex body of knowledge and skill."[19] Once staff nurses become autonomous in their identities, they can extend their field of practice to encompass the expertise of others in the collaborative process. This need to extend themselves led nurses to utilize a new role in nursing.

This new role emerged, contributing to the complexity but effectiveness of the collaborative process. The role of the clinical nurse specialist (CNS) is not a unique entity at the present time. The role and its ultimate influence in planning patient care in the clinical setting has often been discussed in nursing literature. Every CNS probably functions in a different way in various clinical institutions. Initially, each CNS takes a limited caseload of patients and proceeds with care based on expanded educational background in both theory and clinical skills. As the CNS sees the need to extend influence, and as the primary nursing concept is implemented, he or she makes the transition from direct care situations to indirect care situations. "Clinical Nurse Specialists intermittently enter the direct care interface; their impact on actual care rendered is determined in part by their ability to affect the values, thought process and behavior of others and in part by the amount of time they are actually able to spend in the interface."[20] Spending time in the interface process is imperative to developing influence. This interaction can be with the client and family, physicians, other health care professionals, and, of course, nursing—the essential component in the staircase leading to unified structure that Styles identified.

Time given, availability, openness, mutual trust, and respect are all necessary elements for true collaboration between a CNS and a staff nurse.

Miller speaks to these very terms. The consultant needs to develop an air of (1) friendliness; (2) confidentiality, which leads to trust; (3) mutuality in terms of peer effort; (4) resisting resistance by avoiding the temptation to be the savior, thereby shying away from brilliant insights and snap judgments; and (5) an air of coordinating interdependence, thereby influencing professional autonomy.[21]

These components have been related as essential to the milieu of collaboration. Miller's request to avoid the "big play" or "coup" in consultation is a most practical suggestion. In this component, the consultant takes into account the group norms and behaviors. Most group norms should not be continually shattered by sensational new ideas. Consultants have to use their influence in a sensitive and caring manner when dealing effectively with groups. Changes that are adapted to easily in the clinical setting have to come from within the group. The staff must believe that they are essential elements in altering nursing interventions or in promoting the process of change. They need to know that their involvement makes a difference.[22] The CNS can provide, as Peterson describes, "an environment that stimulates the internal drive for motivation."[23] This motivation is needed to develop the self-identity of the nurse. The CNS plays a role in creating a climate that fosters coordinated interdependence and professional autonomy.

The CNS can "provide guidance in applying the nursing process, enhance patient assessment, refine problem definition selection from various nursing interventions, and evaluate the effectiveness of care provided."[24] The CNS interacts with all phases of the nursing process and practice. Thereby, nursing is nursing is nursing. The CNS acts as a catalyst and as a support for nurses' interventions. The CNS can act as a liaison among a variety of health care professionals and departments. The CNS helps to validate and consent. With the background and expertise of the CNS, others can be helped to see the overall outcome of patient care. The CNS can "assist the staff to focus on the long range process of providing nursing care and to avoid becoming overwhelmed by the hour-to-hour stresses of task performance."[25]

Let's explore an example of how this process can work. A young child is burned. Involved in her care are the primary and associate nurses, CNS, student nurse, nurse's aide, physical therapist, school teacher, recreational therapist, the visiting nurse, and, of course, the family. The concern is allowing the patient with major burns to go home. To accomplish this task, the following had to be initiated:

- teaching the patient and the responsible family member the proper care of the burns;
- obtaining costly but needed supplies for a family with limited resources;

- assessing the home situation to rule out environmental needs that would limit successful burn care;
- having both the patient and family learn range-of-motion exercises;
- facilitating the use of positive coping patterns for the patient and her family to use to deal with the terrifying pain during the dressing change;
- developing a plan to help the patient finish the school term despite weeks missed in the classroom;
- encouraging the patient to continue with her developmental task of industry by completing projects in recreational therapy;
- further developing social skills through interaction with other children on the unit and in recreational therapy;
- teaching the need for adequate consumption of protein for burn healing; and
- conveying the importance of the need for follow-up outpatient appointments.

No wonder all these people were needed in the collaborative process!

The CNS had contact with the child in the intensive care unit. She was involved in direct hands-on care during the child's stay in the intensive care unit. Prior to the child's transfer to the surgical nursing unit, the CNS gave a preliminary report to the staff and facilitated the arrangement of a primary nurse. The collaborative process had already begun. Various needs were noted immediately. The need for the family to have financial assistance to care for the child at home and in the hospital was most evident. The extensive burns required the help of the physical therapist. In the realization of the requirement for long-term care, the need to continue this beautiful child's social development was a priority. This would involve the special services of the recreational therapist and the school teacher.

The CNS directed the family to the accounting office to apply for a crippled children's fund to help cover the cost of burn care. Knowing the child could not go to recreational therapy for several days, the CNS approached the recreational therapist to bring projects to the bedside. The school teacher contacted the child on a daily basis. The physical therapist was called by the CNS to intervene in the child's care.

The stage had been set. The CNS, from her initial contact, was best able to assess the overall scope of the child's care and help coordinate the essential elements to meet the various needs. The staff nurse is often so involved with minute-to-minute concerns that she has little time and personal space to visualize the total sphere of care consistently. However, the primary nurse is in the best position to coordinate the child's day-to-day activities while performing daily assessments of the particular needs of the child. The CNS would be available for direct care at times, but at other times the involvement would be more indirect when the CNS dealt with the needs of other patients.

The primary nurse and the CNS performed teaching to both mother and child. Conflict did not exist in this collaborative effort, as consensus in teaching methods was reached in previous collaborative processes. It was imperative that teaching was consistent to ensure successful assimilation of the information. Repeating the same information was not a concern, since repetition is important in the learning process. The CNS, primary nurse, physical therapist, nurse's aide, and student nurse would have daily conferences with mother and child present in the room. The primary nurse, CNS, and physical therapist would document nursing care needs in the kardex and progress notes. By using these effective tools to communicate with each other, conflict over power and control did not arise.

The nurse's aide was used as a facilitator in the time-consuming whirlpool procedure. She collaborated with both the primary nurse and the CNS concerning the utilization of her skills in setting up equipment for the whirlpool room. Teaching for the nurse's aide was directed to her understanding and dealing with the behavioral responses of a child enduring a painful procedure. She incorporated this understanding in her support of the child, as there was an occasional need for the nurse's aide to stay with the patient in the whirlpool room while the nurse checked on her other patients.

The student nurse was also an integral part of the process. She had the luxury of being able to spend time in fostering the child's social skills, as well as to reinforce constantly the teaching she learned from both the primary nurse and the CNS. The collaboration process also incorporated resources in the community, which was necessary to make the process complete. The process would not be complete without the visiting nurses. They went out to the home for a predischarge visit to validate the environmental safety of the home. The CNS was able to follow up with the child in the outpatient setting along with the physical therapist. It is difficult for the primary nurse to be available for outpatient appointments due to her responsibilities in the inpatient setting. This necessitates the need for the CNS to provide feedback on the visit, as well as the child and her family returning to the nursing unit so that others may see the happy results of a coordinated collaborative effort.

It stands to reason that a coordinated collaborative effort is beneficial in containing health care cases. Early planning in arranging primary nurses and resources essential for care enables the most efficient use of health care personnel. Discharge plans that coordinate people and supplies allows families to be prepared to stay out of the hospital once released. Costly emergency room visits and complications can be avoided with health care personnel involved in the collaboration process with other staff in regard to teaching, supplies, and equipment.

"Communication" is the key word in this process of collaboration. The nurses surveyed stated that most of their involvement in the collaborative process took place in informal discussions about clients. Actual consultation also scored highly. More formal involvement in the collaborative process, such as nursing care planning through documentation and care conferences, was equally valued in terms of utilization. This collaboration may be processed in a variety of ways as described from results of the survey. There are the official consultations and nursing care conferences. Those are valuable entities in the collaborative process, but time clouds some of the effectiveness of the outcomes unless the interventions are evaluated continually.

Continual assessment, evaluation, and planning are essential to promoting accurate patient care. The informal process is often utilized as a means to further collaboration. This process involves the visibility of clinical nurse specialists on the nursing unit on a daily basis. With their expertise, they can assess the clinical situation and decide what would benefit from their interventions. However, they cannot proceed alone. The collaborative process is initiated through communication with the staff nurse, whether primary or associate nurse. The CNS who only deals directly with the client and sidesteps the staff nurse will lose out on the benefits of the collaborative process. Fighting over control of the patient must be avoided at all costs. The subject of control within nursing roles has to be clearly established by both parties prior to the real work of collaboration.

Another coordinated collaborative effort can occur when one CNS interfaces with another CNS. A majority of CNSs are linked to a medical diagnosis or service. Some patients are slotted into one physiological domain and thereby deal with one physician and one CNS. However, there are other clients to whom life has dealt a complexity of physiological alterations, thereby requiring several physicians, bringing the client into contact with several CNSs. To meet the client needs without providing confusion, collaboration is sorely needed. Territories need to be respected, but all parties must keep in mind that the client and family are not terribly interested in role variety and functions in nursing.

Again, collaboration starts with communication. This can be done formally or informally. CNS-to-CNS consults are most stimulating to those involved. Both parties can see the long-range goals and needs. Each CNS determines if he or she can help work toward these long-term outcomes or simply be involved in short-term goals. Some CNS expertise may be needed for a short period of time and can be gradually withdrawn when no longer needed. The most consistently involved CNS would be the main coordinator of outcomes. The CNS for general surgery may be involved in the care of a neonate who requires a surgical intervention. He or she would collaborate with the CNS for neonatology to determine the value of his or her interventions. The CNS for general surgery can be involved in short-term goals directed toward surgical recovery, while the CNS for neonatology coordinates the long-range discharge planning.

These two qualified nurses determine their own level of involvement after assessing patient needs. Patient rounds can be instituted on the patients overlapping on clinical services. Each nurse is aware of the need to intervene personally or offer expertise and knowledge to other CNSs. To avoid overloading a client in dealing with a surplus of people, the CNS may opt to stay clear of a family and remain on the fringe of consultation. However, some families can deal with a variety of health care professionals and view involvement by others as a positive intervention in meeting their own goals and outcomes.

The subject of control and role definition relates to the discussion of whether the CNS should be in a staff or line position. There are advocates and proponents for each utilization of the role. With the line position comes power in the reward, expert, legitimate, and even coercive domains. Although CNSs may be able to make more effective changes swiftly in line positions, they may find themselves overloaded with managerial or administrative duties that take them away from patient care. However, the role of the CNS is more clearly defined in a line position. When other health care professionals view the CNS role clearly, they can identify his or her influence or power in various clinical situations. The staff nurse may be more open to change, or perhaps more resistant, if directly accountable to the CNS.

The CNS in the staff position on the organizational chart encounters more role confusion in the clinical setting. Although there are written responsibilities inherent in the role, they are not as clear as in the line position. The CNS in the staff position does not possess the coercive or legitimate power available to those in the line position. He or she is limited to the use of reward, reverent, and expert power. Administrative duties are not so all-encompassing, and this CNS may be more available to the staff nurse. Even though the CNS may be more available, lack of authority over the staff may either limit or increase the CNS's involvement with the staff nurses in the patient care setting.

Drucker has stated that the only way a CNS can do a decent job in a staff position is to (1) genuinely want others to get credit, (2) start out with the aim of enabling others to do what they want to do, (3) have the patience to let others learn rather than do the work themselves, and (4) not abuse the position to manipulate and play favorites.[26] Having the patience to let others learn instead of doing the work oneself is one of the biggest tasks of the CNS. It requires continual collaboration with staff nurses on three shifts who are directly involved in the client's care. This requires planning, time to deal adequately with each nurse, and careful scrutiny during the evaluation process. Staff nurses support interventions of the consultant when they are actively involved in the planning and decision making. Their motivation ebbs when they have to support totally the interventions of a consultant without adequate collaboration.

Staff positions allow the CNS to be approached as a "safe" resource for assistance in problem resolution.[27] Nurses do this constantly, whether the concern is of a personal or clinical nature. The CNS serves as a sounding board for all the day-to-day clinical hassles, and staff nurses can feel that their complaints were told to a safe but somewhat authoritative figure. Staff nurses perceive that the CNS is on the clinical and not the managerial level since few CNSs in the staff position are responsible for evaluating staff nurses. Information shared often helps to develop nurses' identities and thereby gears their developmental stages toward autonomy.

Part of the task of the CNS role is to run interference among a variety of health care professionals. Whether in a staff or line position, the CNS needs to believe that "an individual's success depends on strong social support systems and the knowledge of informal relationships."[28] To reciprocate, the staff nurse can serve as a steadfast supporter of the CNS role and interventions. The staff nurse often communicates to others about the interventions of the CNS in collaboration and can promote the CNS effectively in other collaborative processes with other nurses.

The collaborative process is complex, and the previous discussion has just touched the surface. There is collaboration between staff nurse and staff nurse, staff nurse and CNS, CNS and CNS, staff nurse and CNS with student nurse, and staff nurse and CNS with other ancillary nursing personnel. The collaborative process may begin as a duet, but may quickly multiply to many people.

All efforts do not turn out positively in a collaborative process. At times, the collaborative process fails. There may be a variety of reasons for this. It could be that the collaborators did not agree on specific plans of care. The client and family may not have felt involved in the collaborative plan and thereby did not see the need to comply with the action plan. Sometimes, those in the collaboration have to confront the fact that clients may have enormous physical problems and do not reach the outcomes desired for wellness. Frustration is felt by all when the collaborative process fails to meet its goals. It is important to re-evaluate the process and support those involved instead of looking for places to lay blame.

From consent within the collaborative practice comes a unified policy or plan of action that is agreeable to all parties. The sixth step described by Styles in this staging process is developing a unified structure.[29] If the plan agreed upon in the stage of unified policy can be duplicated easily in a variety of settings, then policies and procedures could evolve, and step six would be completed in establishing unified structures. According to Valentine, Kraus states that the collaborative process is "a cooperative venture based on shared power and authority. It is non-hierarchical in nature. It assumes power based on a knowledge or expertise as opposed to power based on role or role function."[30]

Styles summarizes it well. "Collaboration for its many purposes and in its many forms can be a potent force to achieve our professional aims."[31] These aims can be directed outward from patient care. Many authors allude to the force or power that can come from a unified group of nurses. These nurses must not isolate themselves in their own group, but must branch out in networking and professional groups to reaffirm that nursing is nursing is nursing. "Rather than adding formal, structural network organizations, nurses need to learn networking skills: sharing, trusting, valuing and supporting other nurses."[32] We as nurses should dedicate ourselves to nurturing and providing support to each other as we strive to provide care to our patients and families.

Nursing Administration

"Nursing is what nursing management is all about," states the Patient Care Manager (PCM) for Infectious Disease at St. Louis Children's Hospital. The nursing manager (or supervisor/head nurse as this person is sometimes called) holds a middle management position within the organization. In this position, the manager collaborates in two directions.

In one direction, the manager collaborates with the staff nurses and other unit personnel. The PCM, in commenting on her perceptions of the role, further states, "The manager matches the needs with the resources. This person must be cognizant of the actual as well as potential skills, knowledge, expertise, creativities and other abilities in order to assist the nurse to maximally use these resources." The manager must also be a "doer"; that is, managers must collaborate with and motivate the staff nurse to use the nurse's resources to meet patient/family needs. In order to do this, managers may sometimes use "power" only, i.e., they practically dictate what will be done with, to, and for the patients and their families. Dennis defines "positional power" as ". . . obedience owed to the person because of legitimate power of command vested in the official position." She continues: "The higher ranking the position, the more power its holder wields. The holder of the position therefore has a 'right' to influence his or her subordinates, and the subordinates have an obligation to accept this influence. . . ."[33] However, competent managers usually collaborate with, not dictate to, those with whom they work.

In the same direction, the manager is charged with facilitating the staff nurse's collaboration with patients and their families. This topic is discussed earlier in this book.

In the other direction, the manager collaborates with the nurse executive on more hospital-wide issues. The manager uses the nurse executive for global direction and long-range planning. In addition, the manager models his or her management style after the nurse executive.

While talking to another St. Louis Children's Hospital manager, it was pointed out that this middle manager also collaborates with other middle managers, such as in maintenance and housekeeping. One other way the PCM collaborates with these other departments is through committee work. This PCM states that she is "proactive," that is, she seeks out hospital-wide committees in which she feels patient care representation is needed. She also pointed out that she does not need to go through the nurse executive, but has the freedom to collaborate whenever and wherever she deems appropriate.

While the roots of the consulting/consenting/collaborative process emanate from the "grass roots" of nursing, one has to recognize the integral role of the nurse manager. The manager has to have a link with both the consultee and consultant. Although managers may not be an active part of the collaborative process, their informal as well as formal approval of the collaborative process help ensure credibility in the clinical setting.

The clinical nurse specialist may hold a line or a staff position in any given institution. If a line position is held, frequently the CNS also fulfills the duties of the manager and/or head nurse and therefore collaborates as mentioned earlier. If the CNS holds a staff position, he or she usually works collaboratively with the manager. At St. Louis Children's Hospital, a patient care manager-clinical nurse specialist linkage is being developed. This provides for a formal mechanism in which the manager and specialist work toward improving care for patients and families and increasing utilization of staff resources.

Recently, the PCM/CNS link was utilized to operationalize the concept of "family-centered care," which is found in the mission statement of St. Louis Children's Hospital. The two groups (PCMs and CNSs) met together for a one-day workshop, raised, and then attempted to answer the following questions:

- How is "family-centered care" defined?
- What are the leadership roles in implementing family-centered care (i.e., the role of the PCM, the role of the CNS, the role of the primary nurse), and how will they be evaluated?
- What are the problems inherent in carrying out "family-centered care" at the unit level?
- What other patient care people (such as social workers and chaplains) need to be involved with the concept of "family-centered care"?
- What are the future implications?

A two-hour follow-up meeting was held for the small groups that worked on these items to report to the large group to bring closure to the issue.

"The Nurse Executive's goal is to develop administrative policy which creates an environment that facilitates and enhances the staff nurse's ability to provide patient care in a safe and effective manner," states the Vice President for Patient Care at St. Louis Children's Hospital. She explains that one of the ways she helps to make this happen is by bringing about policy and employee benefits that "facilitate (rather than hinder) staff giving care and practicing professional nursing." The nurse executive collaborates through the managers to staff and ultimately enhances patient/family care. The nurse executive collaborates through the clinical nurse specialist for patient/family care and ultimately staff development. The formal link between manager and clinical specialist, therefore, optimizes quality patient care.

NURSING INTERFACING WITH NURSING IN EDUCATION AND RESEARCH

Collaboration with Nursing Education

Discussion of collaboration in nursing is not complete unless one investigates the relationships and roles of service and education. Which came first? Did implementation precede theory or did a knowledge base of the beginnings of nursing spawn nursing itself?

Historically, it is evident that nursing practice, nursing services, and nursing education were once interwoven. We began in a collaborative mode, but we lost the tie that bound us together. Nursing was striving for a position on a peer level with other health care professionals. To promote this goal, nursing turned to the arenas of higher learning. That was a prudent move. However, in the process, nursing turned away from nursing practice and nursing service instead of incorporating both roles in the educational domain.

The separation of education and service was complete by 1959.[34] At this time, federal funding was delegated to institutions of higher learning and not to nursing services. Nursing suffered some changes in this developmental phase. Nursing educators "lost touch with realities of nursing practice and have lost their credibility both with the students, and with clinicians, in the practice of nursing."[35] With this loss came distrust and loss of mutual respect for each other's contributions to the clinical setting. Problems arose because negative characteristics of individuals usually caused generalization, often formulated in statements that instructors were too ideal and clinically incompetent and that those in nursing service were poor role models.[36] The gap widened between education and service; however, this developmental phase brought the arrival of a new breed of nurses. Now nurses shared educational backgrounds similar to other health care professionals. With added skills and expertise, the nurse gained her self-identity and was able to develop autonomous behavior.

With autonomy came the nurse's ability to question, seek out answers, and to take certain risks regarding nursing practice. This risk-taking bordered on the daring. The nurse was willing to buck the system and to try to alter methods to promote better nursing outcomes. Nurses were able to look at the contribution of others in their same field without losing their own sense of worth. This daring requires "decisiveness and opening oneself to differences of others, viewing those differences as just that—rather than threats or superiority."[37]

The changing nurse was not the sole contributor to the movement directed toward the collaborative mode that once existed previously. There are now enough nurses to do the job, and this has raised competition in the nursing field. University and college campuses have also faced decreased enrollment and increased college costs. The economics of both systems dictate that we must "develop effective, efficient programs maximizing the use of resources."[38] We need to identify and assess resources both in the clinical setting and in the educational setting and see that their uses are maximized. Resources are best utilized in the collaborative mode.

This collaboration should speak to a mutuality of goals. There should be a mutual effort directed toward practice and educational concerns. These goals can be reached when each party shares a similarity in structure, values, and power.[39] The structure is inherent in the organizational framework of the service and academic institutions. Various modes of structural alterations will be discussed later in the chapter. Although structural changes are essential for true collaborative effort, the identification of shared values is the basis for social integration.[40] "Agreement on the essence of nursing is a basis for achieving shared values."[41]

Dealing with the essence of nursing is inherent in all modes of collaborative practice in nursing. Differences can be overcome and obstacles avoided if both parties share the same values regardless of role structure or power. Power and its influence on nursing were previously discussed. Legitimate and coercive power may come with structure, but reverent and expert power are evident when one shares mutual respect and concerns for common goals.

Seeking the fulfillment of common goals calls for the networking of nurses for the collective synthesizing of new images of reality for nursing.[42] One of these images speaks of the need to develop the nurse who can bring traditional values and skills into the patient care arena, which is now shadowed by economic trials and technical miracles. Nursing theory belongs to the laws of applied sciences. These sciences represent "a synthesis of theory from the pure sciences that is unique in the case of each discipline."[43] Obtaining knowledge from the pure sciences allows us to share information that is so important to the collaborative mode.

Utilizing knowledge acquired from nursing and other disciplines is one expectation of the new graduate. Expectations expand to include the ability to assume responsibility and to be self-directed. The nurse needs to analyze and synthesize data that may be conflicting in nature. The nurse has to manage multiple perspectives and be able to take risks when negotiating and/or maintaining the professional role.[44] Such encompassing expectations can be achieved only through the coordination of talent that exists within service and educational institutions.

The literature speaks of the need for this collaboration, and one can state that this process has reached a satisfying status in some institutions. There are affiliation and unification models in existence today. Institutions boast that the nurse executive for patient care also has the title "dean of the school of nursing." There are other settings that have clinical nursing chiefs under the nurse executive to coincide with the medical chiefs responsible for care. These nurses are responsible for the realm of nursing practice, education, and research for faculty, students, and staff. The University of Rochester is involved in a medical center superstructure involving medical staff, administrative representatives, and nursing staff.[45] Nursing has representation on committees concerning planning activities and quality assurance. Nurses form their own self-governing operations.[46]

The clinical teaching assistant is a role that is evident in the scheme of collaboration between education and service. These clinical teaching assistants are primary nurses who carry the dual responsibility of patient care and student teaching. The role is designed to integrate "fragments of nursing practice, education and research into a unified professional nursing practitioner-teacher-researcher role."[47] These nurses work side by side with the practitioner-teacher, who is ultimately responsible for the care given by the students. The practitioner-teacher is involved in teaching the teaching assistant about methodologies utilized in the clinical instructor role. The practitioner-teacher also shares course requirements and objectives with the teaching assistant to ensure consistency in communicating learning needs to the students.[48]

Obviously, there are several role models from which to choose. These various role models of collaboration, affiliation, or unification are described in the literature. However, what percentage of nursing schools and institutions do these statistics cover? What is happening in the majority of institutions committed to nursing education? Surely they must be aware of the growing trend of bridging the gap between education and service. However, is the imagination and administrative backup present that is sorely needed to make changes? What can be done without changes in organizational structure? And, should "emphasis (be) placed on changing nursing schools or hospital structure?"[49] Values can be shared and power manipulated among the roles inherent in nursing service and nursing education. Values can be shared regardless of where the power lies. Once values are shared and commitment is reached, then people in varying roles can open up to each other and avoid the pitfalls in utilizing role power to accomplish the task.

Value sharing is initiated from the commitment to the essence of nursing. What is it that we want to teach new graduates? Should they learn how to change the system encountered in the clinical setting? Let us hope that they are given sufficient knowledge base and guidelines to effect change when it is needed and also to be able to support essential traditional nursing interventions. The utilization of mentorship can make this happen.

The art of mentorship had its beginning in early Greek times and has been utilized inconsistently in the nursing arena. "Nursing is a profession that has a demonstrated serious lack of talented mentors."[50] Schorr has stated that the "transition from diploma to degree education is the alienating factor" in promoting mentorship.[51] At a time when educational differences may divide nursing groups, mentoring would be useful in combining the needs of experienced graduates with younger, more novice nurses. In this way traditional effective nursing guidelines can be maintained while showing a new theoretical knowledge base in nursing.

Creating assignments and planning for the clinical experience commands time and energy from the faculty member. Too often the instructor has to squeeze in assignment-making between lecture sessions and committee meetings. Where is the commitment from the administration for the instructor to have adequate time for this task? Collaborating with the nurse on the unit in making assignments is necessary. However, the instructor should have sufficient time to review the medical record prior to collaboration. Time is also needed to master new equipments and techniques in the clinical setting. It is the instructor's responsibility to learn before leading a student to the patient's bedside. Clinical instructors should prepare for the clinical area with as much intensity as their students.

The process of collaboration between service and education can then begin prior to the students coming to the unit. The staff would appreciate the collaborative process in assignment-making, as this offers them some control and insight into the students' learning through course objectives. The staff also appreciates the student and instructor who are well prepared for caring for their assigned patients. Nursing programs that do not allow sufficient time for student preparation in the clinical area need to be aware of the input this makes in the clinical setting. Although the main goal of the student is to learn, the student should also be a help and not a hindrance in the clinical area. Staff nurses should use guidance in collaboration in care but should not be responsible for teaching unless previous arrangements were made concerning their expanded roles.

There is much discussion concerning the need for faculty practice in the clinical setting. Faculty practice does not simply mean working as a staff nurse in the clinical setting.[52,53] Ford states that Florence Nightingale spoke of activities that are related to faculty input in care: "They must be scholarly in orientation with associated scholarship outcomes and they must have the care of the patient as their central focus."[54] The results of the First Annual Symposium on Nursing Faculty Practice clearly articulated that faculty practice involves roles in service agencies that meet the above criteria. This means involvement in indirect or direct care, staff development, quality assurance, clinical advancement, and various hospital committees. The process of giving direct care does not necessarily mean that the needs for associated scholarship are met.[55]

Meeting the needs of associate scholarship would alleviate the need for the institution to request outside consultation services. The skills of nursing education instructors and administrators could enhance the management background of hospital personnel while promoting an aura of collaboration and a freedom of give and take.

Direct care is an excellent way to refresh clinical skills and to be socially integrated into the hospital system. However, it is not the only way that clinical skills can be mastered. If prepared well for the clinical setting and if varied resources in the hospital setting are utilized, then the instructor must be truly accountable in all aspects of patient care. The instructor can only be accountable through utilization of sound theoretical and clinical skills. The instructor will master clinical skills if truly involved with the care that the students give their patients. Sitting in the conference room grading papers does not reinforce the instructor's collaborative role with the students or staff. The instructor needs to be actively involved with the concerns of the unit.

Involvement and a caring attitude toward the needs of both students and staff speak to the openness essential to the collaborative mode. This openness then leads to the mutual trust and respect that is required in every collaborative setting. Thereby, values and power are shared to bridge the gap between service and education without relying solely on structural changes in the organizational chart. This is not to devalue the influence that structural changes can play in improving the climate for the collaborative mode; rather it is to relate that individual personalities are really the key to the process of collaboration. If the individuals are committed to the need to bring the "collaborative expertise of the professional into a shared relation to achieve the high standards of practice and education," then limitations confronted with structured roles can be overcome.[56] With collaboration, we will have the power to prepare the student adequately for the clinical arena.

Collaboration in planning the education of well-prepared nurses will indeed take time and energy from both institutions of service and education. Outcome will be affected. The student should not require an extensive internship if the quality of instruction was woven with clinical expertise. The cost of orienting new graduates would certainly decline as they could master skills and learn the system easier if they were encouraged to have contact with service personnel. Students certainly feel the lack of clinical expertise and thereby turn to working with minimal supervision in institutions for increased mastery of skills. Surely collaboration between service and education throughout the student's education would alleviate this concern.

Valiga describes what is involved in the training of professionals. The training for uncertainty is what the professional needs to encounter problems evolving from day-to-day practice.[57] With the reality of nursing service and the ideal of nursing education, we should be able to give the professional nurse what is needed to practice adequately in the clinical setting. This collaboration would convey "attitudinal and emotional components such as maintenance of one's self-confidence even when one does not have an answer to the problem, a willingness to take responsibility for key decisions that may rest on only partial information, willingness to make decisions under conditions of high risk, and the ability to inspire confidence in the client even when operating in an area of high uncertainty."[58]

All these abilities can be accomplished only through the collaboration of those in practice with those in the educational setting. Each has to accept the different stressors inherent in each role. Generally, the service nurse has to practice in a fast-paced manner while the clinical instructor has more time to contemplate his or her activities. Naturally, the staff nurse would be client-oriented in the collaborative process. Often it is stated that the clinical instructor is student-oriented. While oriented to the student, the clinical instructor must have the client as the number one priority. It is only by placing the client first that the student can witness that the ideals emanating from the instructor coincide with those of the staff. If the student sees both the staff and instructor place the client's needs above others, then the student truly sees consistency in the practice setting. This by no means states that students should not be fully supported in their endeavors by both faculty and staff. The student will receive more support through the consistent actions of others.

Ford stated that the reward system is different between education and patient care. Those involved with patient care receive immediate rewards from the client or other health care professionals, while the nurse involved in the educational field can experience only long-range rewards from the system.[59]

Sharing concerns and knowledge in the clinical area can bring both reward systems to each party involved in collaboration for increased quality in education. Gilson-Parkevich stated it well—"We all possess talent, expertise and creativity within our individual selves to shape our collective destiny."[60]

Collaboration with Nursing Research

Almost from the beginning, nursing research, once established within the realm of academia, became the sole property of nursing faculty. With the issue of "publish or perish" within university settings, all kinds of research escalated in schools of nursing. Much of this research, called "nursing research," dealt with the study of nurses or with sociological, psychological, or educational variables relative to nurses themselves. Nursing research, because of the varied backgrounds of nurse researchers, actually looked at nurses, students, the educational process, and so forth, with researchers coming from education, sociology, psychology, and the like. Since nurse educators were not necessarily nurse clinicians, very little clinical research was done; that is, the essence of what nurses *do* with patients was not investigated.

More recently, however, "nurse researchers with master's and doctorate degrees are being hired by hospitals, health departments, and other agencies for the specific purpose of doing clinical research directed toward the general goal of improving patient care."[61] Thus, nursing research involving patient care variables is coming to the fore.

In addition, some nursing faculty are seeking clinical appointments, as, for example, in the Case Western Reserve University Program[62,63,64] and the Rush model.[65] Nursing faculty prepared in research now are directing their efforts toward clinical issues, and in this way nursing research is becoming more clinical.

The ANA *Social Policy Statement*[66] mandates collaboration between the nurse researcher and the nurse practitioner when, following a statement on collaboration among nursing and the various other health professionals, it states that "nursing must also recognize . . . relationships within nursing and between nursing. . . ." In addition, a "collective" effort is encouraged through "fostering development of nursing theory, derived from nursing research into those conditions that are the focus of practice, so as to explain observations and guide nursing actions."[67]

Another cause contributing to the issue of generating practice-based research is the matter of professionalism. In recent years, nursing as a profession has been and is being explored. One attribute of a profession is that it must generate its own knowledge base. The knowledge base for nursing generates from clinical practice—consequently, a switch to emphasis on clinical research. From this emphasis stemmed doctorates in nursing with increased specialization and hence more attention to clinical nursing research.

Paralleling clinical nursing research was the focus on the nursing process in both nursing education and nursing service. Padilla speaks to the similarities between the nursing process in terms of problem-solving and evaluation techniques and the research process, which asks significant questions.[68] She believes that the two—nursing process and research process—are so similar that it is relatively easy for the transition to be made from what nursing service is already doing to actually conducting research studies. The rationale she proposes for using nursing research in the clinical setting is that this will allow nurses to use the scientific method to find answers to nursing questions. Some of the uses she advocates are in the area of evaluation, accountability, and cost effectiveness. In addition, research will yield answers that are valid, reliable, and generalizable.

How does one go about initiating a research program in a clinical setting? Padilla took an already existing program—the nursing audit—and transformed it into a research project. "An exciting challenge" is how Chance and Hinshaw[69] describe their work in initiating and maintaining a formal research program in a hospital. They list several requisites. First is the need for a commitment of resources and time from the hospital's nurse executive. This means that the nurse executive believes that research is needed and is willing to find resources that include nurse researchers and provide time for researchers and others to define the studies and carry them out.

Second, any new program takes money. The nurse executive must find the money to fund a research program. This may require innovation or turning another position within the hospital structure into one for research. A nursing research program needs a budget of its own.

Third, the environment must be right. This means that the units within the hospital and their staff are open to having research activities carried out in their areas. One would probably assume that a nursing research program would be most viable in large medical centers where teaching and research of physicians is pervasive. After all, the staff is accustomed to having research activities, and this indeed may be so. But on the other hand, the staff may also be reluctant to have *nursing* research carried out because it is a new phenomenon for them and they may already feel overwhelmed by "research."

In fact, nonteaching hospitals lead us to the fourth issue, and that is that administrators and managers in nonteaching hospitals can encourage outsiders to conduct studies within their institutions. Some sources of outsiders are obviously teaching institutions, i.e., universities that do not have teaching hospitals of their own. Faculty and graduate students could be invited to do studies in these nonteaching hospitals. Nurse executives should have some idea of what kinds of questions they want answered so that when the outsiders come in, they will be meeting the research needs of those institutions also.

Another component of a newly designed research program in any institution is that it follow the overall goals of the nursing department. The aims and objectives of the research program should closely follow those of the department it serves, and the type of research designed initially should help to legitimize the program per se. The initial planning should include ways to maintain the program once it is inaugurated.

Davis describes two mechanisms to legitimize research activities by nurses that imply that nursing administration supports research activities. The first of these is through "released clinical time."[70] Research takes time, and nurses need to be freed from their everyday activities to design and carry out research activities. At St. Louis Children's Hospital we work with Management By Objectives (MBO), and as a part of this we can ask to work toward "innovative goals." One of the contributors to this book planned for and negotiated for released time to work on a research project. Sometimes it takes some creativity on the part of the nurse to negotiate with the administrator for released time to do research. The point is that the nurse does not need to wait for the administrator to offer: the nurse can initiate the request.

Another way that nursing administration legitimizes research, according to Davis, is by recognizing nursing research through the institution's formal reward system. Again, at St. Louis Children's Hospital, by using MBO, the nurse can elect to state research as one of the objectives.

Davis further speaks to "research reference groups." In this way, she gets together nurses who understand and value research and who are committed to furthering the research goals of the institution.

Problems encountered in the clinical setting when research is proposed is the topic of an article by Hinshaw, Chance, and Atwood.[71] They state that it requires real collaboration and negotiation for a research program to work. Among some of the problems one could anticipate is the fact that nurses are not acclimated to research as are persons in other disciplines. Most of the straight sciences, whether behavioral or physical, focus on research and publishing when instructing their students in the discipline. This is not true of nursing. Nurses are taught to "do," and in some instances, not to "think." Thus, the nurse is so busy "doing" that there is no time left for research, and there is very little contact with the research process.

Let us now look at the roles of specific kinds of nurses within a research framework. Until now the assumption is that nurse researchers would design the research and carry it out in any way in which they could.

Just as the nurse executive creates the climate for quality patient care, so too should the administrator create a climate for clinical research. Sylvester speaks to the nursing administrator's responsibilities for research.[72] First, the administrator creates an environment that supports nursing research. One way of doing this is to establish policies and indicate in other ways that research is valued and expected. Second, the administrator provides recognition and rewards for research, for example, funding travel to present research findings at an out-of-town conference. A research budget is the third indicator of administration support for research. Some administrators are hiring researchers to be part of the staff. Included in budgeting is the availability of work time for research activities.

This raises the issue of cost/benefit. The benefits for doing clinical research are many; among them is that nurses will use the scientific method to find answers to nursing questions. Research will yield answers that are valid, reliable, and generalizable. This in turn will facilitate implementation and evaluation of the findings as well as communication of same. In addition, if solutions to the questions are "done right," so to speak, it eliminates "re-inventing the wheel." Solutions will not have to be found again and again.

Ventura, an innovative nursing administrator, used the delphi technique to identify priorities for nursing research.[73] Using administrators, clinical staff, and researchers as a selected panel, sequential questionnaires were distributed to obtain a consensus of opinion while maintaining anonymity of the panel members. This technique avoids confrontation among panel members.

The role of the clinical nurse specialist in research activities is well documented in the literature. Krone and Loomis, in describing the Conduct and Utilization of Research in Nursing (CURN) project, promote using the clinical specialists and outside researchers.[74] By involving clinicians in the project, the probability of their utilizing the findings is increased.

Another role of the CNS involves serving on institutional review boards.[75] By so serving, the CNS becomes aware of nurse involvement in research studies.

Much emphasis is placed in the literature on utilization of research findings in the clinical setting.[76,77] Obviously, it is the task of the CNS to make use of research findings and to facilitate the application of such findings in the clinical setting.

Clinical research questions should come from clinical practice, and who is better able to raise the questions than the CNS? The CNS does not necessarily have to design the research but should be working collaboratively with a nurse researcher to help define the questions. The CNS may also participate in data collection.

Staff nurses, too, should be consulted for the clinical questions, and, like the CNS, they can participate as data collectors.

Lastly, the collaboration between researcher and researcher needs to be addressed. Bergstrom et al. report on a "successful consortium" of seven investigators in four different locations. This collaboration provided a large sample size in a relatively short period of time and maximum use of resources.[78] This was an example of nurse researcher to nurse researcher collaboration. Nurse researchers also need to collaborate with researchers in other disciplines, since nursing is an applied science.

Collaboration between the nurse researcher and the nurse clinician in practice is imperative. Nursing research is a must for the discipline of nursing, but the research questions should come from clinical practice.

SUMMARY

We are all nurses who happen to possess a variety of roles and functions. Some of us have more power than others. Others utilize personal influence to achieve goals. However we deal with the client and family, whether directly or indirectly, we all have an interest in and commitment to the outcomes of patient care. This commitment to the patient and family also needs to be reflected in our concern for each other. We as nurses have to dedicate ourselves as support systems nurturing each other's endeavors. We are all in this together. Our differences in opinion should air our concerns and not divide. No one is going to come to our rescue. We are a force and a power. We can utilize this to facilitate outcomes of care. And, again, we can use this force and power to bring cohesiveness into nursing today.

NOTES

1. Margretta Styles, "Reflections on Collaboration and Unification," *Image*, Winter 1984, p. 21.

2. Barbara Carper, "Fundamental Patterns of Knowing in Nursing," *Advances in Nursing Science*, October 1978, p. 17.

3. American Nurses' Association, *Nursing—A Social Policy Statement* (Kansas City, Mo.: ANA, 1980), p. 7.

4. Ibid., p. 21.

5. Jenniece Larsen, "Nurse Power for the 1980's," *Nursing Administration Quarterly*, Summer 1981, p. 75.

6. J. French and B. Raven, "The Bases of Social Power" in *Studies in Social Power*. D. Cartwright ed. Ann Arbor: Institute of Social Research, University of Michigan, 1970.

7. Margretta Styles, "Reflections on Collaboration and Unification," *Image*, Winter 1984, p. 22.

8. Ibid.

9. Sr. Calista Roy, *Introduction to Nursing: An Adaptation Model*. Englewood Cliffs, NJ, Prentice-Hall, Inc., 1976, pp. 183, 185.

10. A. J. Krakowski, "Psychiatric Consultation in the General Hospital: An Exploration of Resistances." *Diseases of the Nervous System*. 36. May, 1975, pp. 242–244.

11. Linda Norton, "The Clinical Nurse Specialist as Consultant," *Nursing Administration Quarterly*, Fall 1981, p. 71.

12. Marlys Peterson, "Motivating Staff to Participate in Decision Making," *Nursing Administration Quarterly*, Winter 1983, p. 67.

13. Chris Kasch, "Interpersonal Competence and Communication in the Delivery of Nursing Care," *Advances in Nursing Sciences*, January 1984, p. 72.

14. Kathryn Chance, "Nursing Models: A Requisite for Professional Accountability," *Advances in Nursing Science*, January 1982, p. 58.

15. Linda Miller, "Resistance to the Consultation Process," *Nursing Leadership*, March 1983, p. 11.

16. Ibid., p. 13.

17. Claudette Varricchio, "The Process of Influencing Decisions," *Nursing Administration Quarterly*, Summer 1982, p. 10.

18. Ibid.

19. Priscilla McKoy, "Interdependent Decision Making: Redefining Professional Autonomy," *Nursing Administration Quarterly*, Summer 1983, p. 26.

20. Lois Johnson et al., "A Model of Participatory Management with Decentralized Authority," *Nursing Administration Quarterly*, Fall 1983, p. 40.

21. Linda Miller, "Resistance to the Consultation Process," *Nursing Leadership*, March 1983, p. 14.

22. Marlys Peterson, "Motivating Staff to Participate in Decision Making," *Nursing Administration Quarterly,* Winter 1983, p. 64.

23. Ibid.

24. Mary Blount et al., "Extending the Influence of the Clinical Nurse Specialist," *Nursing Administration Quarterly,* Fall 1981, p. 59.

25. Ibid.

26. P. Drucker, *Management—Tasks, Responsibilities, Practices.* New York, New York, Harper and Row, 1974.

27. Mary Blount et al., "Extending the Influence of the Clinical Nurse Specialist," *Nursing Administration Quarterly,* Fall 1981, p. 61.

28. Janice Meisenhelder, "Networking and Nursing," *Image,* October 1982, p. 77.

29. Margretta Styles, "Reflections on Collaboration and Unification," *Image,* Winter 1984, p. 22.

30. Patricia Valentine, "How Does Your Unit Operate?," *Nursing Leadership,* June 1983, p. 41.

31. Margretta Styles, "Reflections on Collaboration and Unification," *Image,* Winter 1984, p. 22.

32. Janice Meisenhelder, "Networking and Nursing," *Image,* October 1982, p. 79.

33. Karen Dennis, "Nursing's Power in the Organization: What Research Has Shown," *Nursing Administration Quarterly,* Fall 1983, p. 48.

34. Ann Marriner, "Unification of Nursing Education and Service," *Nursing Administration Quarterly,* Fall 1983, p. 59.

35. Marjorie Batey, "Structural Consideration for the Social Integration of Nursing," in *Structure to Outcome: Making it Work,* ed. Kathryn Barnard (Kansas City, Mo.: American Academy of Nursing, 1983), p. 2.

36. Ibid., p. 7.

37. Tamar Gilson-Parkevich, "Stepchildren in the Family: Aiming Toward Synergy Between Nursing Education and Service—From the Nursing Service Perspective," in *Structure to Outcome: Making it Work,* ed. Kathryn Barnard (Kansas City, Mo.: American Academy of Nursing, 1983), p. 39.

38. Ibid., p. 33.

39. Marjorie Batey, "Structural Consideration for the Social Integration of Nursing," in *Structure to Outcome: Making it Work,* ed. Kathryn Barnard (Kansas City, Mo.: American Academy of Nursing, 1983), p. 8.

40. Ibid., p. 6.

41. Ibid.

42. Tamar Gilson-Parkevich, "Stepchildren in the Family: Aiming Toward Synergy Between Nursing Education and Service—From the Nursing Service Perspective," in *Structure to Outcome: Making it Work,* ed. Kathryn Barnard (Kansas City, Mo.: American Academy of Nursing, 1983), p. 39.

43. Lucille Joel, "Stepchildren in the Family: Aiming Toward Synergy Between Nursing Education and Service—From the Faculty Perspective," in *Structure to Outcome: Making it Work,* ed. Kathryn Barnard (Kansas City, Mo.: American Academy of Nursing, 1983), p. 44.

44. Theresa Valiga, "Cognitive Development, A Critical Component of Baccalaureate Nursing Education," *Image,* Fall 1983, p. 116.

45. Loretta Ford, "Organizational Perspectives on Faculty Practice: Issues and Challenges," in *Structure to Outcome: Making it Work,* ed. Kathryn Barnard (Kansas City, Mo.: American Academy of Nursing, 1983), p. 17.

46. Ibid.

47. Mary Clark, "Staff Nurses as Clinical Teachers," *American Journal of Nursing,* February 1981, p. 314.

48. Ibid., p. 315.

49. Robert Allison, "Nursing Unification in Principal Teaching Hospitals," *HCM Review,* Summer 1981, p. 55.

50. M. Hamilton, "Mentorhood: A Key to Nursing Leadership," *Nursing Leadership,* March 1981, p. 4.

51. T. Schorr, "The Lost Art of Mentorship," *American Journal of Nursing,* November 1978, p. 1873.

52. Loretta Ford, "Organizational Perspectives on Faculty Practice: Issues and Challenges," in *Structure to Outcome: Making it Work,* ed. Kathryn Barnard (Kansas City, Mo.: American Academy of Nursing, 1983), p. 14.

53. Lucille Joel, "Stepchildren in the Family: Aiming Toward Synergy Between Nursing Education and Services—From the Faculty Perspective," in *Structure to Outcome: Making it Work,* ed. Kathryn Barnard (Kansas City, Mo.: American Academy of Nursing, 1983), p. 49.

54. Loretta Ford, "Organizational Perspectives on Faculty Practice: Issues and Challenges," in *Structure to Outcome: Making it Work,* ed. Kathryn Barnard (Kansas City, Mo.: American Academy of Nursing, 1983), p. 13.

55. Ibid., p. 14.

56. Marjorie Batey, "Structural Consideration for the Social Integration of Nursing," in *Structure to Outcome: Making it Work,* ed. Kathryn Barnard (Kansas City, Mo.: American Academy of Nursing, 1983), p. 3.

57. Theresa Valiga, "Cognitive Development: A Critical Component of Baccalaureate Nursing Education," *Image,* Fall 1983, p. 116.

58. Ibid.

59. Loretta Ford, "Organizational Perspectives on Faculty Practice: Issues and Challenges," in *Structure to Outcome: Making it Work,* ed. Kathryn Barnard (Kansas City, Mo.: American Academy of Nursing, 1983), p. 26.

60. Tamar Gilson-Parkevich, "Stepchildren in the Family: Aiming Toward Synergy Between Nursing Education and Service—From the Nursing Service Perspective," in *Structure to Outcome: Making it Work,* ed. Kathryn Barnard (Kansas City, Mo.: American Academy of Nursing, 1983), p. 39.

61. Elaine Larson, "Combining Nursing Quality Assurance and Research Programs," *Journal of Nursing Administration,* November 1983, p. 32.

62. Rozella M. Schlotfeldt and Jannetta MacPhail, "An Experiment in Nursing," *American Journal of Nursing,* 69, no. 5 (May 1969).

63. Ibid.

64. Ibid.

65. Luther Christman and J. P. Lysaught, "A Luther Christman Anthology," *Nursing Digest* 11, no. 2.

66. American Nurses' Association, *Nursing—A Social Policy Statement* (Kansas City, Mo.: ANA, 1980), p. 7.

67. Ibid., p. 8.

68. Geraldine V. Padilla, "Incorporating Research in a Service Setting," *Journal of Nursing Administration*, January 1979, p. 44.

69. Helen C. Chance and Ada Sue Hinshaw, "Strategies for Initiating a Research Program," *Journal of Nursing Administration*, March 1980, p. 32.

70. Marcella Z. Davis, "Promoting Nursing Research in the Clinical Setting," *Journal of Nursing Administration*, March 1981, p. 22.

71. Ada Sue Hinshaw, Helen C. Chance, and Jan Atwood, "Research in Practice: A Process of Collaboration and Negotiation," *Journal of Nursing Administration*, February 1981.

72. Donna C. Sylvester, "Nursing Administration's Responsibilities for Research," *AORN Journal* 31, no. 5 (April 1980): 850.

73. Marlene R. Ventura and Barbara Waligora-Serafin, "Setting Priorities for Nursing Research," *Journal of Nursing Administration*, June 1981, p. 30.

74. Kathleen P. Krone and Maxine E. Loomis, "Developing Practice-Relevant Research: A Model that Worked," *Journal of Nursing Administration*, April 1982, p. 38.

75. Eileen C. Hodgman, "Research Policy for Nursing Services: Part 1," *Journal of Nursing Administration*, April 1981, p. 31.

76. Elizabeth A. Hefferin, JoAnne Horsley, and Marlene R. Ventura, "Promoting Research-Based Nursing: The Nurse Administrator's Role," *Journal of Nursing Administration*, May 1982.

77. Cheryl Stetler, "Research Utilization: Defining the Concept," *Image: The Journal of Nursing Scholarship*, pp. 40–44, Spring 1985, Vol. XVII, No. 2.

78. Nancy Bergstrom et al., "Collaborative Nursing Research: Anatomy of a Successful Consortium. *Nursing Research*, Vol. 33, No. 1, pp. 20–25, January/February 1984.

SUGGESTED READINGS

Allison, Robert. "Nursing Unification in Principal Teaching Hospitals." *HCM Review*, Summer 1981, pp. 55–61.

American Academy of Nursing. *Structure to Outcome: Making it Work*. Kansas City, Mo.: American Academy of Nursing, 1983.

American Nurses' Association. *Nursing—A Social Policy Statement*. Kansas City, Mo.: ANA, 1980.

Bailey, Katherine, and Swenson-Feldman, Elizabeth. "Innovative Approach to the Nursing Process." *Nursing Administration Quarterly*, Spring 1982, pp. 71–76.

Batey, Marjorie. "Structural Consideration for the Social Integration of Nursing." *Structure to Outcome: Making it Work*. Edited by Kathryn Barnard. Kansas City, Mo.: American Academy of Nursing, 1983, pp. 1–11.

Beck, Cheryl. "The Conceptualization of Power." *Advances in Nursing Science*, January 1982, pp. 1–17.

Benoliel, J. Q., and Berthold, J. S. *Human Rights Guidelines for Nurses in Clinical and Other Research*. St. Louis, Mo.: American Nurses' Association (Publication No. D-46, 5M, 7/75), 1975.

Bergstrom, Nancy, et al. "Collaborative Nursing Research: Anatomy of a Successful Consortium." *Nursing Research* 33, no. 1 (January/February 1984): 20–25.

Blount, Mary, et al. "Extending the Influence of the Clinical Nurse Specialist." *Nursing Administration Quarterly*, Fall 1981, pp. 53–62.

Braack, Lucy, and Cate, Marcella. "Collaborative Research Promotes Patient Teaching." *Nursing Administration Quarterly* 4, no. 2 (Winter 1980): 97–100.

Carper, Barbara. "Fundamental Patterns of Knowing in Nursing." *Advances in Nursing Science*, October 1978.

Chance, Kathryn. "Nursing Models: A Requisite for Professional Accountability." *Advances in Nursing Science*, January 1982, pp. 57–65.

Chance, Helen C., and Hinshaw, Ada Sue. "Strategies for Initiating a Research Program." *Journal of Nursing Administration*, March 1980, pp. 32–39.

Chater, Shirley. "Faculty Practice Considerations in Academic Health Centers' Schools of Nursing." *Structure to Outcome: Making it Work.* Edited by Kathryn Barnard. Kansas City, Mo.: American Academy of Nursing, 1983, pp. 59–65.

Clark, Mary. "Staff Nurses as Clinical Teachers." *American Journal of Nursing*, February 1981, pp. 314–318.

Crabtree, Mary. "Effective Utilization of Clinical Specialists within the Organizational Structure of Hospital Nursing Service." *Nursing Administration Quarterly*, Fall 1979.

Davis, Marcella Z. "Promoting Nursing Research in the Clinical Setting." *Journal of Nursing Administration*, March 1981, pp. 22–27.

Dean, Patricia G. "Facilitating Research." *Nursing Management*, May 1982, pp. 23–24.

Dennis, Karen E. "Nursing's Power in the Organization: What Research Has Shown." *Nursing Administration Quarterly* 8, no. 1 (Fall 1983): 47–57.

Flaherty, M. Josephine. "Perspectives in Nursing: Nursing Managers and Nursing Research." *Supervisor Nurse*, June 1980, pp. 64–65.

Ford, Loretta. "Organizational Perspectives on Faculty Practice: Issues and Challenges." *Structure to Outcome: Making it Work.* Edited by Kathryn Barnard. Kansas City, Mo.: American Academy of Nursing, 1983, pp. 13–29.

Gilson-Parkevich, Tamar. "Stepchildren in the Family: Aiming Toward Synergy Between Nursing Education and Service—From the Nursing Service Perspective." *Structure to Outcome: Making it Work.* Edited by Kathryn Barnard. Kansas City, Mo.: American Academy of Nursing, 1983, pp. 31–41.

Gilliss, Catherine. "Collaborative Practice in the Hospital: What's in it for Nursing." *Nursing Administration Quarterly*, Summer 1983, pp. 37–44.

Hamilton, M. "Mentorhood: A Key to Nursing Leadership." *Nursing Leadership*, March 1981, pp. 4–13.

Hefferin, Elizabeth A.; Horsley, JoAnne; and Ventura, Marlene R. "Promoting Research-Based Nursing: The Nurse Administrator's Role." *Journal of Nursing Administration*, May 1982, pp. 34–41.

Hinshaw, Ada Sue; Chance, Helen C.; and Atwood, Jan. "Research in Practice: A Process of Collaboration and Negotiation." *Journal of Nursing Administration*, February 1981, pp. 33–38.

Hodgman, Eileen C. "Research Policy for Nursing Services: Part 1." *Journal of Nursing Administration*, April 1981, pp. 30–33.

Joel, Lucille. "Stepchildren in the Family: Aiming Toward Synergy Between Nursing Education and Service—From the Faculty Perspective." *Structure to Outcome: Making it*

Work. Edited by Kathryn Barnard. Kansas City, Mo.: American Academy of Nursing, 1983, pp. 43–57.

Johnson, Lois, et al. "A Model of Participatory Management with Decentralized Authority." *Nursing Administration Quarterly,* Fall 1983, pp. 30–46.

Kasch, Chris. "Interpersonal Competence and Communication in the Delivery of Nursing Care." *Advances in Nursing Sciences,* January 1984.

King, Joan. "Nursing Action Research: Using Clinical Nurse Instructors." *Nursing Administration Quarterly,* Summer 1982, pp. 47–51.

Kramer, M. "Collegiate Graduate Nurses in Medical Center Hospitals." *Nursing Research* 18, no. 3 (1969): 196–210.

Kramer, M. "Role Conceptions of Baccalaureate Nurses and Success in Hospital Nursing." *Nursing Research* 19, no. 5 (1970): 428–439.

Krone, Kathleen P., and Loomis, Maxine E. "Developing Practice-Relevant Research: A Model that Worked." *Journal of Nursing Administration,* April 1982, pp. 38–41.

Kuhn, Janet. "An Experience with a Joint Appointment." *American Journal of Nursing,* October 1982, pp. 1510–1571.

Larsen, Jenniece. "Nurse Power for the 1980's." *Nursing Administration Quarterly,* Summer 1982, pp. 74–82.

Larson, Elaine. "Combining Nursing Quality Assurance and Research Programs." *Journal of Nursing Administration,* November 1983, pp. 32–35.

LeBreton, Preston P. "Determining Creativity Strategies for a Nursing Service Department." *Nursing Administration Quarterly,* Spring 1982, pp. 1–11.

Marriner, Ann. "Unification of Nursing Education and Service." *Nursing Administration Quarterly,* Fall 1983, pp. 58–64.

McKoy, Priscilla. "Interdependent Decision Making: Redefining Professional Autonomy." *Nursing Administration Quarterly,* Summer 1983, pp. 21–29.

Meisenhelder, Janice. "Networking and Nursing." *Image,* October 1982, pp. 77–80.

Miller, Linda. "Resistance to the Consultation Process." *Nursing Leadership,* March 1983, pp. 10–15.

Morton, Paula. "The Financial Distress of Higher Education: Impact on Nursing." *Image,* Fall 1983, pp. 102–106.

Murphy, Shirley, and Hoeffer, Beverly. "Role of the Specialties in Nursing Science." *Advances in Nursing Science,* July 1983, pp. 31–39.

Norton, Linda. "The Clinical Nurse Specialist as Consultant." *Nursing Administration Quarterly,* Fall 1981, pp. 69–74.

Notkin, Marilyn. "Collaboration and Communication." *Nursing Administration Quarterly,* Fall 1983, p. 29.

Nyberg, Jan. "The Role of the Nursing Administrator in Practice." *Nursing Administration Quarterly* 6, no. 4 (Summer 1982): 67–73.

Padilla, Geraldine V. "Incorporating Research in a Service Setting." *Journal of Nursing Administration,* January 1979, pp. 44–49.

Peterson, Marlys. "Motivating Staff to Participate in Decision Making." *Nursing Administration Quarterly,* Winter 1983, pp. 63–68.

Pilette, Patricia. "Caution: Objectivity and Specialization May Be Hazardous to Your Humanity." *American Journal of Nursing,* September 1980, pp. 1588–1590.

Pilette, Patricia. "Mentoring: An Encounter of the Leadership Kind." *Nursing Leadership,* June 1980, pp. 22–26.

Roux, Rose. "Communication and Influence in Nursing." *Nursing Administration Quarterly,* Spring 1978, pp. 51–57.

Schlotfeldt, Rozella M., and MacPhail, Jannetta. "An Experiment in Nursing." *American Journal of Nursing* 69, no. 5 (May 1969).

Schlotfeldt, Rozella M., and MacPhail, Jannetta. "Experiment in Nursing: Implementing Planned Change." *American Journal of Nursing* 69, no. 7 (July 1969).

Schorr, T. "The Lost Art of Mentorship." *American Journal of Nursing,* November 1978, p. 1873.

Styles, Margretta. "Reflections on Collaboration and Unification." *Image,* Winter 1984, pp. 21–23.

Styles, Margretta. "Who's Who Among Nursing Leaders." *Nursing Leadership,* June 1983, pp. 61–66.

Sylvester, Donna C. "Nursing Administration's Responsibilities for Research." *AORN Journal* 31, no. 5 (April 1980): 850–855.

Varricchio, Claudette. "The Process of Influencing Decisions." *Nursing Administration Quarterly,* Summer 1982, pp. 8–15.

Valentine, Patricia. "How Does Your Unit Operate?" *Nursing Leadership,* June 1983, pp. 40–43.

Valiga, Theresa. "Cognitive Development: A Critical Component of Baccalaureate Nursing Education." *Image,* Fall 1983, pp. 115–119.

Ventura, Marlene R., and Waligora-Serafin, Barbara. "Setting Priorities for Nursing Research." *Journal of Nursing Administration,* June 1981, pp. 30–34.

Werner, June. "Joint Endeavors: The Way to Bring Service and Education Together." *Nursing Outlook,* September 1980, pp. 546–547.

Chapter 7

Nurses and Clients as Collaborators

Valann Tasch, R.N., M.S.N., C.P.N.P.

INTRODUCTION

Collaboration between the client and the health professional has developed slowly. The idea is based on Western society's democratic ideals and was given impetus by the consumer movement. More recently, the focus on cost effectiveness in the health care field further supports the need to collaborate with the client to promote health and self-care abilities. The high cost of health care services and the use of prospective payment and capitation for reimbursement for services to hospitals has brought about a renewed emphasis on the need for the client to become more knowledgeable about health-promoting practices and to assume a more active role in managing existing health problems. Various theories and models that have been developed to explain health and sick-role behaviors and research on factors associated with compliance with therapeutic regimens provide additional support for the value of developing collaborative relationships with clients.

In this chapter, various theories and models will be described, and some of the findings from compliance research that lend support for collaborative relationships with clients will be reviewed. The implications that these models and research findings have for practice will also be discussed.

THEORIES AND MODELS
SUPPORTING COLLABORATION

The Concept of Locus of Control

The concept of locus of control is derived from Rotter's social learning theory, which is used to help explain why people behave in certain ways.

Rotter notes, "In its most basic form, the general formula for behavior is that the potential for a behavior to occur in any specific psychological situation is a function of the expectancy that the behavior will lead to a particular reinforcement in that situation and the value of that reinforcement."[1] In other words, persons will be more likely to do something if they expect that a desired goal will be achieved as a result. How much the particular goal is valued is also an important factor.

For example, whether an adolescent boy will take medication on a regular basis to control his seizures will depend on whether he expects that taking medication will produce seizure control and on how much he values seizure control as a reinforcement or outcome. It may be that he views taking medication as a symbol of abnormality emphasizing his differentness from peers. The reinforcement or outcome may therefore need to be reframed to become more relevant for the adolescent boy who seeks to be like his peers. For example, he may be more likely to take his medication if he knows that he will need to be seizure-free for a period of time in order to obtain a driver's license.

In elaborating on the concept of locus of control, Rotter describes individuals as having an external locus of control or as having an internal locus of control. He states,

> An individual who is described as having a belief in external control of reinforcement perceives reinforcement following some action of his own, but not entirely contingent upon his action. It typically is perceived as the result of luck, chance, fate, under control of powerful others, or as unpredictable. An individual who has a belief in internal control of reinforcement perceives reinforcement as contingent upon his own behavior or his own relatively permanent characteristics.[2]

In other words, individuals with an external locus of control orientation think that they have little control over what happens to them, that outcomes are controlled by powerful others, are unpredictable, or occur purely by chance. Individuals with an internal locus of control, on the other hand, think that they have control over outcomes and actively seek to achieve desired outcomes.

To use again the example of the adolescent boy, if he has an external locus of control orientation, he might believe that complete seizure control is principally a matter of luck or chance. He may therefore rationalize that since complete seizure control is more a matter of luck or chance and since taking medication only serves to emphasize his differentness from peers, there is little reason to take medication on a regular basis. On the other hand, the adolescent boy with an internal locus of control may recognize that while he may not have total control over the desired outcome of complete seizure control, there are things he can do to increase the likelihood that the desired outcome will occur, that is, take his medication on a regular basis.

Although one's expectation that certain behaviors will bring about certain outcomes is considered a major determinant of behavior potential in social learning theory, it is considered only one of three major determinants. The second is the extent one values the outcome or reinforcement, and the third is the psychological situation.[3]

Studies support the relevance of considering an individual's locus of control orientation in facilitating the development of positive health and sick-role behaviors. For example, Strickland, in her review of research on internal-external locus of control expectancies and health attitudes and behaviors, noted that those individuals with an internal locus of control expectancy attempted to maintain their physical well-being and to guard against accidents and disease to a greater extent than individuals who held external locus of control expectancies. In addition, those individuals with an internal locus of control expectation who valued their health sought more information about health maintenance, and when stricken with a disorder appeared to learn more about the disease.[4]

Studies also suggest that behavior change is enhanced when programs are geared to an individual's locus of control orientation. In a study by Auerback et al., it was found that patients responded differently to specific and general presurgery information depending on their locus of control orientation. According to dentist ratings, individuals with an internal locus of control did better in surgery after receiving specific information about the procedure and sensations they might expect. They adjusted poorly in surgery after receiving general, marginally relevant material about the dental procedure. The reverse was true for patients with an external locus of control.[5,6]

In a study by Wallston et al., it was found that clients with an external locus of control orientation lost more weight in an externally oriented group program, while clients with an internal locus of control orientation lost most weight in an internally oriented self-directed program.[7] It is noted that an internally oriented program should provide more choice of treatment, more involvement of the patient making choices, and a strong emphasis on individual responsibility. An externally oriented program might focus on increasing the belief that health can be controlled and on providing social support to improve health-related practices.[8]

In general, there is support for considering a client's generalized expectancy that certain behaviors will bring about certain outcomes or reinforcement. Research indicates that whether a particular individual acquires positive health and/or sick-role behaviors will depend, in part, on our ability to adapt our approach to the individual's particular locus of control orientation.

A collaborative relationship would be essential to achieving this goal. One needs to get to know the client and her or his locus of control orientation and values to determine useful approaches to acquiring desired outcomes. For example, the nurse might help a client with an internal locus of control orientation explore alternative approaches to achieving desired outcomes. In addition, the nurse might support the client's efforts to obtain needed information, skills, services, and other social supports and to make necessary adjustments to prevent or minimize the impact of disease on functioning.

A more explicit approach to assisting an individual with an internal locus of control orientation would be contracting. Behavior modification principles are based on operant conditioning, which notes that the probability that a behavior will occur is increased when the behavior is followed by a rewarding stimulus known as positive reinforcement. A behavior is decreased if it is followed by punishment or if it is ignored. Contracting involves collaboration between the client and health care provider to determine what health behaviors are desired and what changes need to take place to achieve these behaviors. In addition, reinforcers for the desired behaviors must be determined by the client.

Since major changes in behavior generally take place slowly over time, the resultant plan for a particular client/family may include a series of contracts, each building on successful accomplishment of the previous contract. Each contract specifies the behavior to be performed and the reinforcement desired. It is signed by both the health care provider and the client, indicating agreement to the terms.

Contracts can be useful also when working with clients with an external locus of control orientation. By setting up a contract that facilitates accomplishment of a desired goal, clients can begin to learn that they can have control over outcomes. In addition, the collaborative relationship that is established can be a source of social support to provide additional encouragement to alter certain behaviors.

The following two examples will illustrate the use of contracting in the clinical setting. Steckel describes the use of contracting with hypertensive patients. In looking at a specific example of a hypertensive patient, she noted that six health-related behaviors needed to occur to achieve compliance with his medical regimen. The client needed to take daily medication, keep regular clinic appointments, lose 15 pounds, stop smoking, reduce on-the-job stress, and exercise regularly. The client identified losing weight as the behavior he wanted to focus on initially. To assist the client in taking the first step toward achieving this goal, a contract was set up to begin eliminating one piece of bread at each meal. The first contract called for him to make a written record each time he eliminated one piece of bread at a meal and to bring this record to the office in three weeks. The reinforcer for this behavior was an early morning medical appointment. The next contract would depend on the client's performance on the previous one and might involve increasing the number of food items that were eliminated or reduced.[9]

Contracts can also be set up with clients/families in the inpatient setting. For example, Anne was a 15-year-old pregnant, developmentally disabled girl hospitalized for management of pre-eclampsia. She was moderately mentally handicapped, but had no physical limitations. The hospital staff was having difficulty managing many of Anne's behaviors. She would strike out at staff members, go into other patients' rooms and disturb them, spit out her medications, and refuse to stay in bed.

Since bedrest was considered crucial for management of her condition, this behavior was focused on first. A baseline evaluation was done to determine the frequency of out-of-bed behavior. In addition, positive reinforcers were determined for Anne. These were determined by observing and talking with Anne and speaking with significant others, including her school teacher. It was noted during this time that Anne would sit with her feet up if someone sat with her. Spending time with an adult was therefore determined to be a positive reinforcer.

A contract was then set up with Anne. She was told that she needed to rest in bed or sit in the wheelchair with her feet up. Initially she would be requested to do this four times per day for a ten-minute time period. When obtaining baseline information it was noted that Anne could be encouraged to sit for ten minutes. The ten-minute time period was therefore considered to be an achievable goal. While Anne was resting in bed or sitting in a wheelchair with her feet up, reinforcers such as records to listen to, coloring books and crayons, cosmetics, and the attention of an adult were to be provided. As a result of these interventions, Anne began to spend more time resting.

It is difficult to determine what variables had the greatest impact on Anne's behavior. Was it the reinforcers? Was it the clear messages to Anne regarding expectations for her behavior? Was it the fact that Anne was given a measure of control over what happened to her? Although it was clear that she needed to rest, she could choose where she rested and what reinforcers she received. Was it the fact that the nursing staff had begun to develop a collaborative relationship with Anne by making an effort to understand her world and her needs and making efforts to accomplish health-related goals within this framework? Was it the development of mutual trust and caring as an integral part of the relationship? I suspect that all these factors interacted in a dynamic fashion to achieve the outcome.

In any case, both of these examples illustrate how contracting can assist clients to develop or maintain an internal locus of control orientation by helping them to achieve behaviors and reinforcers through their own action. For those who already have a strong internal orientation, contracting emphasizes the client's participation and responsibility for health-related behaviors. For those who have an external locus of control orientation, contracting may help them learn that they can have control over outcomes. In addition, the collaborative relationship can be a source of social support to alter certain behaviors.

The Health Belief Model

The Health Belief Model was formulated by Rosenstock et al., and was derived from the social-psychological theory of Lewin. His theory postulated that behavior depended on the value placed by an individual on a particular outcome and the individual's estimate of the likelihood that a given action will result in that outcome. Utilizing this model it is postulated that an individual's readiness to take action relative to a particular health condition is determined by several factors:

1. the individual's perceived susceptibility or vulnerability to the condition,
2. the individual's perceptions of what the consequences would be if the condition would be contracted,
3. the individual's estimate of the action's potential benefits in reducing actual or perceived susceptibility and/or severity weighed against the cost of the proposed action, including the work involved in taking action.[10]

In other words, whether an individual carries out a preventive health measure depends on the person's belief in susceptibility to the condition, the individual's perceptions of what the consequences would be if the condition was contracted, and the action's potential for reducing susceptibility or severity of the condition weighed against the cost of the proposed action.

For example, although dentists advocate daily brushing and flossing of teeth to prevent dental caries and gum disease, this may not be carried out. It may be that a particular individual does not perceive that she or he is vulnerable to problems or does not perceive dental caries or dental disease as severe enough problems to warrant taking the time to brush the teeth on a regular basis.

Although originally formulated to explain preventive health behaviors, others have modified the Health Belief Model to include factors that influence sick-role behaviors. Becker has considered the following additional factors:

1. When considering susceptibility, added dimensions are the individual's belief in the accuracy of the diagnosis, the estimate of resusceptibility, and the individual's subjective feelings of vulnerability to various other diseases or to illness in general.
2. Utilizing the results of compliance research, Becker grouped additional variables into a number of categories among which are demographic, structural, attitudes, and interaction. The only demographic variable associated with noncompliance and medication errors was extremes of age. He noted that in general, compliance is not consistently related to sex, intelligence, education, or marital status.[11]

Haynes noted that the results of clinic-based studies suggested that demographic features of those who continued to attend clinic appointments were not associated with compliance patterns. He concluded that the effect of demographic factors appeared to be much greater on access to health services than on compliance with therapy among patients already in the system.[12]

The structural category includes cost, duration, complexity, side effects, accessibility of the regimen, and the need for new patterns and behavior. Haynes reviewed 185 articles on compliance and noted that regimens that require more extensive behavior change, those that continue over time, and those that are complex reduce compliance.[13] For example, the hypertensive patient described earlier needed to take daily medication, lose 15 pounds, stop smoking, reduce on-the-job stress, and exercise regularly. To achieve these goals would require a number of changes in life style. The client would need to be convinced that the long-range benefits in terms of health status outweighed the costs in terms of changes in life style.

Attitudes include satisfaction with the visit, physician, other staff, clinic procedures, and facilities. Korsch et al., in a study of 800 patient visits to the walk-in clinic of Children's Hospital of Los Angeles, found a number of factors that contributed significantly to patient dissatisfaction—lack of warmth and friendliness on the part of the doctors, failure to take into account the patient's concerns and expectations from the medical visit, lack of clear-cut explanations concerning diagnosis and causation of illness, and use of medical jargon.[14] Studies show positive correlations between patient satisfaction and compliance.[15] These findings also illustrate the importance of a collaborative relationship for patient satisfaction and compliance. These patients valued the quality of the physician/patient relationship and clearly wanted to be active participants in their own care.

Interaction for the most part refers to the doctor-patient relationship. As noted above, the quality of the relationship between the physician and the patient was important for patient satisfaction with care. Haynes noted that studies indicated a positive association between the degree of supervision and compliance.[16]

In examining research considering various components of the Health Belief Model, Becker notes support for the relationship between compliance and perception of susceptibility, severity, benefits, and costs.[17] However, how one might modify health beliefs in relation to behavior is not well studied. The complexity of the issue is well recognized. People have innumerable beliefs, and which ones will have the greatest impact on behavior at any given time is not easily determined; and, as has been noted, there are many factors influencing any specific behavior.[18]

Haynes reviewed articles that reported the testing of a clinical maneuver intended to improve compliance. He classified strategies for improving compliance into educational, behavioral, or a combination of the two. Educational strategies are those that attempt to improve compliance through the transmission of information about a disease and its treatment to patients. Behavior-oriented methods focus more directly on behaviors involved in compliance. They include attempts to reduce barriers to compliance, such as cost and complexity of regimen; to cue or stimulate compliance; and to reward and reinforce compliance. It was found that behavioral and combined strategies were more successful in improving both compliance and therapeutic outcomes than educational strategies alone.[19]

Contracting is a good example of a behavioral strategy used to improve compliance. In the case of the patient with hypertension, the nurse sought to help the client to begin taking steps toward achievement of a long-range goal. By breaking down achievement of the goal into manageable steps, the "costs" in terms of altering behavior became less overwhelming. Through contracting, the client became an active participant in his own care, identifying a goal that was of most value to him. In addition, building in rewards for achievement of desired goals provided additional motivation for change.

From the foregoing discussion, the Health Belief Model and research on compliance support the value of establishing a collaborative relationship between health care provider and client. Factors affecting compliance can best be explored within the context of a collaborative relationship. It is within this context that the nurse can determine how a client perceives a particular illness and how a particular medical regimen is perceived in terms of its benefits to the client in light of the "costs." It is through this relationship also that the nurse can discover and take into account the client's concerns and expectations.

By utilizing this information, the nurse can clarify misconceptions. In addition, the nurse can assist the client in determining how a therapeutic regimen can best be incorporated into the client's life, emphasizing the benefits and minimizing the costs. The process would include the nurse sharing knowledge and assisting the client to develop necessary skills to carry out health care measures.

To illustrate this process further, Susan is an eight-year-old profoundly retarded girl with a seizure disorder. When the nurse met Susan and her mother, Susan had behavior problems that the mother and the school teacher were having difficulty managing. Susan would have outbursts of screaming and aggressive behavior during which she would bite and hit other children. In addition, Susan was having infrequent seizures, with drug levels indicating noncompliance with medication. In speaking with the mother, the nurse discovered that the mother did not understand that medication needed to be given every day to maintain a therapeutic blood level to prevent seizures from occurring. In addition, Susan's behavior was more of a problem to the mother than Susan's seizures.

Interventions included both educational and behavioral strategies. The nurse focused on educating the mother on why medication needed to be given on a regular basis. In addition, she assisted the mother in making a plan as to how she would do this. The mother then became an active participant in planning, with a stake in the outcome. Various approaches were explored, and the one that could best be incorporated into the family's daily routine was chosen. A pill-reminder container was utilized, and medication was to be given in the morning when Susan got up and at bedtime.

The nurse then focused on the biggest problem of concern to the mother, Susan's behavior. The nurse pointed out an observation that the teachers at school had made regarding Susan's behavior: her behavior improved when she was receiving medication on a regular basis. In addition, the nurse referred the mother to the social worker to assist the mother in developing skills in behavior management techniques. To remove a barrier to keeping the appointments with the social worker, arrangements were made to provide transportation for these visits.

As a result of these interventions, medication was given on a regular basis as reflected by therapeutic drug levels. In addition, Susan's outbursts of screaming and aggressive behavior decreased in frequency. Susan's mother became more comfortable in handling Susan. She now had an effective plan for dealing with Susan's behavior.

What factors contributed to these outcomes? After discussing the purpose of regular administration of medication with Susan's mother, the nurse defined the benefits of giving the medication regularly in terms of an outcome valued by the mother—improved behavior. She removed barriers to action by assisting the mother determine what she would do to ensure regular administration of medication and by assisting her to keep appointments with the social worker. This was all done in the context of a collaborative relationship in which both the nurse and the mother shared their knowledge and concerns and determined goals and how they would be met. In terms of the relationship, she demonstrated respect for the mother as an individual by valuing what she had to say and making a plan within the context of the mother's defined needs and priorities.

The Family Crisis Framework

Reubin Hill conceptualized a framework of family crisis that is widely used in family stress research. It is as follows: A (the event and related hardships) interacting with B (the family crisis-meeting resources) interacting with C (the definition the family makes of the event) produce X (the crisis). The course of family adjustment involves a period of disorganization, an angle of recovery, and a new level of organization.[20]

Factors that affect a family's adjustment to stressors are a part of the family's crisis-meeting resources and include the following: personal resources, family system's internal resources, social support, and coping strategies.[21] Personal resources refer to the financial, educational, health, and psychological characteristics that assist in coping with stress. Among characteristics labeled as psychological, one's self-esteem and sense of control over one's life have been identified as personal resources that can reduce the consequences of stress.[22]

Family system characteristics that support effective functioning of the family and individual members has not been thoroughly studied. Lois Pratt studied whether a certain structural pattern described as the "energized family" enabled families to function effectively in support of their members' health. They looked at the level of health and illness, the quality of personal health practices, and the extent and appropriateness of use of professional medical services. They interviewed 273 families in a northern New Jersey city. They found support for their hypothesis. The following are characteristics of the energized family:

1. All members interact with each other regularly in a variety of contexts.
2. Members maintain varied and active contacts with other groups and organizations.
3. Members actively attempt to cope and master their lives.
4. Family tends to be fluid in internal organization (role relationships are flexible, power is shared).

5. Relationships tend to support personal growth and to be responsive and tolerant.
6. Members have a high degree of autonomy within the family.[23]

Social support alleviates or mediates the effect of stress. In citing various studies that looked at the effect of social support on recovery from illness and compliance, Cobb noted that a high level of social support accelerated or facilitated recovery. He described three components of social support:

1. Emotional support, leading recipients to believe that they are cared for and loved;
2. Esteem support, leading recipients to believe that they are esteemed and valued;
3. Network support, leading recipients to believe that they have a defined position in a network of communication and mutual obligation.[24]

In addition, in reviewing 41 articles, Cobb noted that social support was associated with compliance over 80 percent of the time.[25]

Coping strategies are the things that people do to deal with life problems. Pearlin and Schooler note three major types of coping: "These are:

1. responses that change the situation out of which a strainful experience arises;
2. responses that control the meaning of the strainful experience after it occurs, but before the emergence of stress; and
3. responses that function more for the control of stress itself after it has emerged."[26]

In evaluating the results of a study investigating the social origins of personal stress using scheduled interviews with a sample of 2,300 people representative of the population in an urbanized area of Chicago, Pearlin and Schooler noted that the variety of responses and resources one can bring to bear in coping with life strains may be more important in preventing emotional stress than any single coping element.[27] They judged the effectiveness of coping behavior on how well it prevented life's problems and hardships from resulting in emotional stress.[28]

In working with families under stress, it is clear that a number of questions must be considered. How does a particular family view an event? Is the event one that has produced a great deal of tension and disorganization in the family? What changes have occurred in the family as a result of the event? What does the family see as problems? What have they done so far to deal with them? What do they want help with? What other stresses is the family experiencing?

If the family is in crisis, one would help the family to recognize the relationship between the precipitating event and the present crisis state. This helps to clarify the problem and to assist the family to focus directly on the present situation.[29] In addition, one may want to encourage family members to express their feelings about the situation to reduce tension and to help them deal with their feelings. If the crisis event is the diagnosis of a chronic or terminal disease in a family member, the nurse would focus on helping the family members to understand the disease and its management and the implications of this for the future functioning of the family and its members. The family can then be helped to identify various approaches they could take to deal with the various problems identified. Parents of a handicapped child must deal with the crisis precipitated by the birth of an imperfect child. They are faced with the task of adjusting to this fact and its implications for the future growth and development of the child, other family members, and the family itself. The following case study illustrates the importance of a collaborative relationship in working with families under stress.

Mr. and Mrs. Johnson are in their mid-twenties and have high school educations. Mr. Johnson is a farmer, and Mrs. Johnson is primarily a housewife. She works part-time at a family-owned restaurant. Linda is five years old, the product of a twin pregnancy whose twin was stillborn. Linda developed seizures at six months of age, characterized by a fall with gagging and swallowing movements lasting seconds to minutes. These were difficult to get under control. Developmentally, she functions at the two-to-three-year-old level in terms of motor skills. However, she has no speech and follows only simple commands. The cause of her problems is unknown. Linda has a eighteen-month-old brother who developed necrotizing entero-colitis at birth. A colostomy was performed initially, and he subsequently had a pull-through operation with multiple readmissions to the hospital for management of diarrhea and dehydration. He is thought to be normal in cognitive ability.

At the time the nurse met the family, they were focused on control of Linda's seizures, as they hoped that control of seizures would bring about improvement in Linda's speech and language development. Linda was about three years old at the time, and the discrepancy between her motor abilities and speech and language development was less marked. The youngest boy, Tommy, was not born as yet.

In assessing this family, the nurse noted that the family had a number of resources. The parents were healthy and actively working together to meet the family's physical needs. They brought Linda to the clinic regularly for management of her seizures and expressed interest in learning more about Linda's problems and how to manage them. Their main source of social support was the paternal grandparents. In regard to coping strategies, Mr. and Mrs. Johnson were actively attempting to deal with Linda's problems but lacked the knowledge, skills, and support they needed to cope effectively with their situation.

The nurse noted a number of problems. Although the family was able to provide for their physical needs, their economic situation was marginal. In addition, multiple trips to the hospital interfered with the father's ability to get the daily farming chores done. The role relationships between the parents were rigid, leaving much of the burden of caring for the children on Mrs. Johnson. However, this was offset to some degree by the support given by the paternal grandmother. Also, Mrs. Johnson received little emotional support from her husband, as communication between them was limited. The family's hope that achieving good seizure control would alter Linda's developmental progress was unrealistic. In addition, the parents had little time to meet their own needs.

Since the family identified improved seizure control and assistance with developmental stimulation as priorities for them, a plan was made with the physician for an approach to seizure management. In addition, the nurse referred the family to a local center where a multidisciplinary team would evaluate Linda and assist the family to obtain appropriate community services for her, including appropriate school programming. The nurse also hoped that through the center the family would receive the support they needed as they began to understand Linda's limitations and their implications for her future development and functioning.

However, the birth of the younger brother interrupted these plans, and the nurse concentrated on providing support to the family through this difficult period. During this time, the father continued his farming as much as possible, the grandparents cared for Linda, and the mother spent most of her time at the hospital with Tommy. The nurse's main focus was on supporting the family in their attempts to deal actively with their situation, including spending a great deal of time listening as they attempted to come to terms with it.

It was during this period that the mother related that she did not receive enough support from her husband in dealing with Linda's problems. She thought that her husband was aware of the severity of Linda's developmental deficits, but could not admit it. Over time, the nurse had been able to help the mother come to an understanding and acceptance of Linda's limitations, but she had not been able to work with the husband because of his inability to attend clinic on a regular basis. In addition, Mrs. Johnson brought up a number of issues that she had not resolved from an early period in her life. The nurse referred Mrs. Johnson for counseling to assist her to deal with these issues and her relationship with her husband.

In an attempt to incorporate the father more into Linda's management, efforts were made to arrange the clinic appointments so that both could attend more often. It was hoped that that would encourage more communication between the parents regarding Linda's problems. To provide additional social support, the parents were referred to a local parent support group. In addition, Mrs. Johnson was encouraged to think of her own needs and to plan time for herself.

As a result of the collaborative relationship that the nurse was able to develop with this family, the Johnsons were able to cope with multiple stresses without being overwhelmed by them. The nurse's interventions were based on her assessment of the family's personal and family resources, their sources of social support, and coping strategies. In addition, her interventions were based on the family's perception of their situation and their identified needs and priorities. The nurse sought to support the family's coping efforts by helping them to develop plans for dealing with the various needs identified, providing needed information about their children's problems and their management, assisting them to develop needed skills to manage the problems, introducing them to other sources of support, encouraging more open communication, and supporting their efforts in meeting their own needs.

There are many different theories of nursing that have been developed to guide nurses in practice. Regardless of the specific theory, however, the nurse-client relationship is considered central to the achievement of the purposes of nursing. As pointed out by Perlman:

> Relationship is a major motivator of a person's acting, thinking, and feeling in some different ways . . . when I know that you feel with me, that you care about me, that you understand what my reasons and reactions are, then I am more likely to care about you, to want your approval, to listen to you, to take your hope and encouragement into myself and to open my mind to your suggestions or opinions.[30]

Trust, empathy, and caring are essential components of a helpful (and collaborative) relationship. Trust in a relationship enables the client to share concerns, feelings, and hopes more openly and can be fostered by the nurse's own trusting attitude, consistency, reliability, and honesty. For example, in the case of the client with hypertension, if the nurse had not fulfilled her part of the contract, there would have been little chance for trust to develop in the relationship and for the contract to succeed. In the case of Anne, if rewards had not been provided, there would have been little chance that Anne would develop trust in the staff and for the plan to succeed. Anne needed the security of knowing that her world was predictable and individuals could be counted on to do what they said they would do. If this had not happened, Anne would have become more anxious and even less able to cope with her environment.

Empathy, "the ability to enter into the life of another person, to accurately perceive his current feelings and their meanings," enhances understanding between the nurse and the client, enabling the nurse to respond to the client in a more effective and therapeutic manner.[31] Inherent in both components is an attitude of caring or love defined by Hagerman as "a response to others in a manner that expresses awareness and respect for a person as an individual, with knowledge and consideration for his specific needs. . . ."[32]

It is through the relationship that is developed between the nurse and client/family that they come to feel comfortable about sharing their values, beliefs, perceptions, and expectations, thus enabling the nurse to help them to identify their needs and ways they might meet them. It is through this relationship also that the nurse can assist the client/family to acquire and to develop the necessary knowledge and skills to cope with their situation. In addition, it is through this relationship that the nurse can provide the necessary support to the client/family as they strive to learn and cope productively with their situation.

How a particular nurse works with a client/family depends on the nurse's own unique personality and the theories he or she uses to guide his or her practice. To illustrate the use of a collaborative relationship in providing nursing care using one of the nursing theories, I will briefly describe the nursing theory of Dorothea Orem and how this might be used in practice.

Dorothea Orem sees an individual as an integrated whole with varying degrees of self-care ability. Self-care is defined as "the practice of activities that individuals initiate and perform on their own behalf in maintaining life, health, and well-being."[33] The purpose of nursing is to enhance self-care ability. To do this, the nurse and the client come to an agreement about what nursing is required and what will be provided. The nurse may do those things for the client that cannot be done without help. The nurse may guide or support the client in taking desired action. The nurse may provide information or teach new skills or create an environment that fosters self-care abilities.[34]

As an example, Mary and John Smith were expecting their first child. The nurse met them and their new son on the day following delivery. She explained to them that she was a pediatric nurse practitioner and worked with the pediatrician they had chosen to provide for Jeffrey's medical care needs. She related that she would be seeing them and Jeffrey for some of his visits for well-baby and well-child care and would be available by telephone to answer any questions or deal with any concerns they might have about Jeffrey. The new parents related that they had done a great deal of reading about infant care and early development but had many questions about various aspects of care. They wondered if the nurse could be present when they gave Jeffrey his first bath. Following discussion, Mary and John and the nurse identified what things the nurse could be helpful with. The nurse would assist Mary with breast-feeding. In addition, she would help the parents to develop the skills they needed to provide for Jeffrey's needs at home. Being aware of common problems that parents experience in caring for newborns, the nurse planned a time when she and the parents could get together again so that she could answer any questions they had and provide anticipatory guidance.

By establishing a collaborative relationship in which the parents and nurse explore the parents' need for nursing care and together determine how these might best be met, an environment for fostering the development of self-care abilities is created.

CONCLUSION

The models and research presented provide support for considering the uniqueness of the individual client/family—their beliefs, values, and perceptions and the personal, family, and community contexts in which they are functioning—if one wants to help them achieve optimum health. In examining the various examples presented, it is apparent that one could use one or parts of all the models described in working with the client/family. Using Orem's theory of nursing as an overall framework, one can examine the use of other theories as a means of helping the client/family to achieve optimum self-care ability.

If one uses the concept of locus of control, one's focus would be to determine a client's generalized expectancy as to whether certain behaviors will bring about certain outcomes or reinforcement. Approaches could then be geared to the individual's locus of control orientation. Among other things, contracting could be used to assist clients with internal locus of control orientation to maintain a feeling of control over outcomes by emphasizing their participation in and responsibility for their own care. Contracting can provide the structure and support needed to achieve desired outcomes for clients with an external locus of control orientation. At the same time, achieving outcomes or reinforcers through their own action may help individuals learn that they can have control over outcomes. These interventions would foster self-care ability.

If one uses the Health Belief Model, one would explore the client's perception of how a particular illness might affect the client's life. The nurse would also explore the client's perception of the therapeutic regimen in terms of its benefits in the light of the costs. The nurse might then clarify misconceptions or help the client to determine how a therapeutic regimen could best be incorporated into the client's life in a way that the perceived benefits outweighed the costs. Contracting can be seen here as a behavioral strategy to make the therapeutic regimen more manageable and as a means of stimulating and rewarding compliance with the regimen. Ultimately, the goal is to assist the client to develop self-care ability.

If one uses the framework of family crisis, one's goal would be to help the client/family to cope effectively with stress. This might include helping them to gain a sense of control over what is happening to them by helping them to understand the situation and their reactions to it, educating them about a particular disease and its management, helping them to explore various approaches to dealing with the problems identified and helping them to incorporate a particular therapeutic regimen into their lives in a way that the perceived benefits outweighed the costs. In addition, the nurse can help the client/family to identify and use various social supports. The nurse can support actively the constructive coping effort. The nurse's overall focus is to provide the help needed to facilitate the development of optimum self-care ability.

Regardless of one's orientation, the key vehicle for assisting the client and family to achieve their goals is the collaborative relationship. It is through the collaborative relationship that the nurse creates an environment in which optimum health and functioning are an expectation. The goal of the relationship is to identify and provide the knowledge, skills, guidance, and support needed. Whether this goal is achieved depends not only on consideration of specific characteristics of the client/family, but on the quality of the relationship itself.

NOTES

1. Julian B. Rotter, "Some Problems and Misconceptions Related to the Construct of Internal Versus External Control of Reinforcement," *Journal of Consulting and Clinical Psychology* 43, no. 1 (1975): 57.

2. Julian B. Rotter, "Generalized Expectancies for Internal Versus External Control of Reinforcement," *Psychological Monographs* 80 (1, whole no. 609) (1966): 1.

3. Julian B. Rotter, "Some Problems and Misconceptions Related to the Construct of Internal Versus External Control of Reinforcement," *Journal of Consulting and Clinical Psychology* 43, no. 1 (1975): 58.

4. Bonnie R. Strickland, "Internal-External Expectancies and Health Related Behaviors," *Journal of Consulting and Clinical Psychology* 46, no. 6 (1978): 1192–1211.

5. S. M. Auerbach et al., "Anxiety, Locus of Control, Type of Preparatory Information, and Adjustment to Dental Surgery," *Journal of Consulting and Clinical Psychology* 44 (1976): 809–818.

6. Bonnie R. Strickland, "Internal-External Expectancies and Health Related Behaviors," *Journal of Consulting and Clinical Psychology* 46, no. 6 (1978): 1192–1211.

7. Barbara S. Wallston et al., "Development and Validation of the Health Locus of Control (HLC) Scale," *Journal of Consulting and Clinical Psychology* 44 (1976): 580–585.

8. Barbara Strudler Wallston and Kenneth A. Wallston, "Locus of Control and Health: A Review of the Literature," *Health Education Monographs* 6, no. 2 (Spring 1978): 107–117.

9. Susan B. Steckel, "When Patient 'Willpower' Fails, a Written Contract May Succeed," *Consultant*, October 1982, pp. 129–137.

10. Lois A. Maiman and Marshall H. Becker, "The Health Belief Model: Origins and Correlates in Psychological Theory," *Health Education Monographs* 2, no. 4 (Winter 1974): 336–353.

11. Marshall H. Becker, "Sociobehavioral Determinants of Compliance," in *Compliance With Therapeutic Regimens,* ed. David L. Sackett and R. Brian Haynes (Baltimore, Md.: Johns Hopkins University Press, 1976), pp. 40–50.

12. R. Brian Haynes, "A Critical Review of the 'Determinants' of Patient Compliance With Therapeutic Regimens," in *Compliance With Therapeutic Regimens,* ed. David L. Sackett and R. Brian Haynes (Baltimore, Md.: Johns Hopkins University Press, 1976), pp. 26–39.

13. Ibid.

14. Barbara M. Korsch, Ethel K. Gozzi, and Vida Frances, "Gaps in Doctor-Patient Communication," *Pediatrics* 42, no. 5 (November 1968): 855–871.

15. Marshall H. Becker, "Sociobehavioral Determinants of Compliance," in *Compliance With Therapeutic Regimens,* ed. David L. Sackett and R. Brian Haynes (Baltimore, Md.: Johns Hopkins University Press, 1976), pp. 40–50.

16. R. Brian Haynes, "A Critical Review of the 'Determinants' of Patient Compliance With Therapeutic Regimens," in *Compliance With Therapeutic Regimens,* ed. David L. Sackett and R. Brian Haynes (Baltimore, Md.: Johns Hopkins University Press, 1976), p. 35.

17. Marshall H. Becker, "Sociobehavioral Determinants of Compliance," in *Compliance With Therapeutic Regimens,* ed. David L. Sackett and R. Brian Haynes (Baltimore, Md.: Johns Hopkins University Press, 1976), pp. 40–50.

18. John P. Kirscht, "Research Related to the Modification of Health Beliefs," *Health Education Monographs* 2, no. 4 (Winter 1974): 455–469.

19. R. Brian Haynes, "Strategies for Improving Compliance: A Methodologic Analysis and Review," in *Compliance With Therapeutic Regimens,* ed. David L. Sackett and R. Brian Haynes (Baltimore, Md.: Johns Hopkins University Press, 1976), pp. 69–82.

20. Reubin Hill, *Families Under Stress* (New York: Harper & Row Publishers, 1949).

21. Hamilton I. McCubbin et al., "Family Stress and Coping: A Decade Review," *Journal of Marriage and the Family,* November 1980, pp. 855–870.

22. Ibid., p. 861.

23. Lois Pratt, *Family Structure and Effective Health Behavior—The Energized Family* (Boston, Mass.: Houghton Mifflin Company, 1976).

24. Sidney Cobb, "Social Support and Health Through the Life Course," in *Family Stress, Coping, and Social Support,* ed. Hamilton I. McCubbin, A. Elizabeth Cauble, and Joan M. Patterson (Springfield, Ill.: Charles C Thomas Publisher, 1982), p. 189.

25. Ibid., pp. 194–195.

26. Leonard I. Pearlin and Carmi Schooler, "The Structure of Coping," in *Family Stress, Coping, and Social Support,* ed. Hamilton I. McCubbin, A. Elizabeth Cauble, and Joan M. Patterson (Springfield, Ill.: Charles C Thomas Publisher, 1982), p. 115.

27. Ibid., p. 129.

28. Ibid., p. 119.

29. Sally Felgenhauer Baird, "Crisis Intervention Strategies," in *High Risk Parenting,* ed. Suzanne Hall Johnson (Philadelphia, Pa.: J. B. Lippincott Company, 1979), pp. 299–311.

30. Helen H. Perlman, "The Helping Relationship," in *Relationship: The Heart of Helping People* (Chicago, Ill.: University of Chicago Press, 1979), p. 51.

31. B. Kalisch, "What Is Empathy?," *American Journal of Nursing* 73 (1973): 1548.

32. Z. Hagerman, "The Patient Who Is Unable to Love," *Nursing Clinics of North America* 4 (1969): 691.

33. Dorothea E. Orem, *Nursing: Concepts of Practice* (New York: McGraw-Hill Book Company, 1980), p. 35.

34. Dorothea E. Orem, *Nursing: Concepts of Practice* (New York: McGraw-Hill Book Company, 1980).

SUGGESTED READINGS

Arakelian, Maureen. "An Assessment and Nursing Application of the Concept of Locus of Control." *Advances in Nursing Science* 3 (1980): 25–42.

Auerbach, S. M.; Kendall, P. C.; Cutler, H. F.; and Levitt, N. R. "Anxiety, Locus of Control, Type of Preparatory Information, and Adjustment to Dental Surgery." *Journal of Consulting and Clinical Psychology* 44 (1976): 809–818.

Baird, Sally F. "Crisis Intervention Strategies." In *High-Risk Parenting.* Edited by Suzanne Hall Johnson. Philadelphia, Pa.: J. B. Lippincott Company, 1979, p. 299.

Becker, Marshall H. "Sociobehavioral Determinants of Compliance." In *Compliance With Therapeutic Regimens,* Edited by David L. Sackett and R. Brian Haynes. Baltimore, Md.: Johns Hopkins University Press, 1976, p. 40.

Cobb, Sidney. "Social Support and Health Through the Life Course." In *Family Stress, Coping, and Social Support.* Edited by Hamilton I. McCubbin, A. Elizabeth Cauble, and Joan M. Patterson. Springfield, Ill.: Charles C Thomas Publisher, 1982, p. 189.

Hagerman, Z. "The Patient Who Is Unable to Love." *Nursing Clinics of North America* 4 (1969): 664.

Haynes, R. Brian. "A Critical Review of the 'Determinants' of Patient Compliance With Therapeutic Regimens." In *Compliance With Therapeutic Regimens.* Edited by David L. Sackett and R. Brian Haynes. Baltimore, Md.: Johns Hopkins University Press, 1976, p. 26.

Haynes, R. Brian. "Strategies for Improving Compliance: A Methodologic Analysis and Review." In *Compliance With Therapeutic Regimens.* Edited by David L. Sackett and R. Brian Haynes. Baltimore, Md.: Johns Hopkins University Press, 1976, p. 69.

Hill, Reubin. *Families Under Stress.* New York: Harper & Row Publishers, 1949.

Kalisch, B. "What Is Empathy?" *American Journal of Nursing* 73 (1973): 1548–1552.

Kirscht, John P. "Research Related to the Modification of Health Beliefs." *Health Education Monographs* 2 (1974): 455–468.

Korsch, Barbara M.; Gozzi, Ethel K.; and Francis, Vida. "Gaps in Doctor-Patient Communication." *Pediatrics* 42 (1968): 855–871.

McCubbin, Hamilton I.; Cauble, A. Elizabeth; and Patterson, Joan M., eds. *Family Stress, Coping, and Social Support.* Springfield, Ill.: Charles C Thomas Publisher, 1982.

Maiman, Lois A., and Becker, Marshall H. "The Health Belief Model: Origins and Correlates In Psychological Theory." *Health Education Monographs* 2 (1974): 336–353.

Orem, Dorothea E. *Nursing: Concepts of Practice.* New York: McGraw-Hill Book Company, 1980.

Pearlin, Leonard I., and Schooler, Carmi. "The Structure of Coping." In *Family Stress, Coping, and Social Support.* Edited by Hamilton I. McCubbin, A. Elizabeth Cauble, and Joan M. Patterson. Springfield, Ill.: Charles C Thomas Publisher, 1982, p. 109.

Perlman, Helen H. "The Helping Relationship." In *Relationship: The Heart of Helping People.* Chicago, Ill.: University of Chicago Press, 1979, p. 51.

Pratt, Lois. *Family Structure and Effective Health Behavior—The Energized Family.* Boston, Mass.: Houghton Mifflin Company, 1976.

Rotter, Julian B. "Generalized Expectancies for Internal Versus External Control of Reinforcement." *Psychological Monographs* 80 (1, whole no. 609) (1966).

Rotter, Julian B. "Some Problems and Misconceptions Related to the Construct of Internal Versus External Control of Reinforcement." *Journal of Consulting and Clinical Psychology* 43 (1975): 56–67.

Steckel, Susan B. "When Patient 'Willpower' Fails, a Written Contract May Succeed." *Consultant,* October 1982, pp. 129–137.

Strickland, Bonnie R. "Internal-External Expectancies and Health Related Behaviors." *Journal of Consulting and Clinical Psychology* 46 (1978): 1192–1211.

Sundeen, Sandra J.; Stuart, Gail W.; Rankin, Elizabeth D.; and Cohen, Sylvia A. *Nurse-Client Interaction.* St. Louis, Mo.: The C. V. Mosby Co., 1981.

Wallston, Barbara S., and Wallston, Kenneth A. "Locus of Control and Health: A Review of the Literature." *Health Education Monographs* 6 (1978): 107–117.

Chapter 8

Nurses Interfacing with Other Members of the Team

Anne T. Richardson, R.N., M.S.N.

INTRODUCTION

Frequently the word "team" is used to denote a group of people purposefully working together. Chaska defines a team as two or more people with diverse skills in such an association.[1] Yet one needs to look at the "working" or "associated" component to understand the real significance of the concept of the team. It needs to be said that just because people work jointly, they do not necessarily function as a team.

So what are the significant elements that influence team functioning? Are there guidelines that can be used to enhance team interaction?

This chapter will look at a more in-depth definition of team, and will review the purposes, participants, barriers, positive influences, and possible outcomes of this very complex concept.

WHAT PURPOSE DOES A TEAM SERVE?

If one chooses a profession such as art, one would not need a team to meet the identified outcomes of providing a given individual with a profession and producing a commodity or service (e.g., paintings). Maybe one could argue that to be an artist one needs supplies, buyers, promoters, and so on, and therefore is working with others. However, is this a team? Health care offers a very different situation. The needs of patients and families with health problems require numerous professions: physicians, nurses, social workers, secretaries, laboratory, x-ray, pharmacists, chaplains, outpatient services, housekeeping, maintenance, accounting, physical therapy, respiratory therapy, and many more. Obviously a client is also needed. The very nature of the situation mandates that more than a single individual or profession be involved.

But what is a team? Are all involved individuals team members? Can one simply use the definition that states that two or more people working together constitute a team? No. However, I propose that a team approach is a very effective model in providing health care. In fact, it is essential since one discipline cannot meet all needs of patients and families of patients with health problems. An interdependent, interdisciplinary team is required. As Pluckhan states, "the alternative to working together is working alone, which is totally unrealistic in today's society."[2] So since no health care profession can be effective in isolation, a working relationship has to be established.

Actually, there is much in the literature about the positive outcomes of teamwork. The following is not meant to cover it all, but to give the reader the view that the efforts to accomplish true teamwork are worthwhile.

All concerned serve to gain from good team interaction. One major outcome is that mutual goal attainment becomes the focus that allows for collaborative, cooperative, joint activities. This is in contrast to an incompatible, competitive, power status oriented model of functioning. The former allows for complementary roles to evolve, which will result in contributions from each member for which they are best suited.[3] Maximum utilization of knowledge and skills can be gained.[4] The open exchange of information, opinions, and feelings will become the norm from which communication, problem solving, decision making, and planning can flow.[5] It should serve to set the stage for growth of all members by each being able to enjoy the knowledge and evaluational input of others; hence, skills should develop more rapidly.[6] It would also allow for the ability of team members to utilize each other constructively and decrease pressures and stresses that naturally occur (especially pressures that one feels if working on one's own and feeling the need to be responsible for all things).[7] Such communication would also eliminate duplication of efforts. This ultimately benefits both the involved professionals as well as the patients and their families in effort, stress, and cost.

Many benefits can be seen by the patient when team functioning exists: expediency and well-planned actions, a sense of cohesiveness of the caretakers, which provides security, less miscommunication and misdirected facts, and so on. Teamwork lends itself to greater understanding of all regarding the realistic expectations of each other's roles.[8] The criteria for job satisfaction (recognition, challenge, responsibility, and opportunity for growth) can then be addressed—"bringing out the best in the job brings out the best in the employee."[9] Health provision can then be viewed as a cooperative and harmonious process.[10] The whole process of allowing mutual decision making implies mutual respect, which enhances growth, especially of those team members who might view themselves as lower status members.[11,12]

WHAT IS A TEAM?

Gillies discusses group dynamics and begins by saying that a group is "an entity consisting of several individuals having a collective perception of their unity and a tendency to act in a unified manner toward their environment."[13] This definition adds many needed factors to describe a team.

Gillies goes on to say that all objectives of such group functioning fall into one of two categories: (1) the achievement of some special goal or task, or (2) the maintenance or strengthening of the group itself.[14] Both components are equally relevant.

The first category actually can be broken down into three areas when discussing health care teams: (1) the goal of providing an occupation for individuals, (2) the goal of providing a needed service, and (3) the specific tasks or activities that go into providing that service. Some health care professionals have been known to fear that giving up specific tasks will threaten their occupation. Often professionals define their jobs in specific and narrow ways and then proceed to provide a service based on that definition without recognizing that the provider's and consumer's needs may be different. The issue of how various professions view their jobs will be looked at further, but I would render a guess that the demise of any job opportunity in health care will be determined more by the effectiveness of services rather than by the obsolescence of any given profession. In our present society the need for services seems to be growing rather than narrowing, but that should not be confused with the issue of individual job satisfaction.

So often discussions occur about various tasks that different professions perform. The delineation of tasks will be covered further in the chapter, but here I would like to just look at the overall problem of defining teamwork by using the limited definition of people simply working together. To illustrate, let's say a patient is hospitalized for hypertension. Working together might be described as the physician writing orders for the administration of an antihypertensive medication, the pharmacy providing it, the nurse administering it, and the patient swallowing it with the outcome of lowered blood pressure readings. These are all task-related activities to achieve a specific goal, and all these people are working together for the same goal. However, the question is: do the physician, nurse, pharmacist, and patient function as a team? Some might say yes. However, the limited nature of this teamwork should be apparent. By Gillies' definition and criteria, not until the component of relationship maintenance is introduced does a true team emerge.[15]

One certainly has heard this phenomenon referred to in sports, too. One may have a collective body of highly skilled and trained athletes, but unless they work together in a certain manner one will not hear those people say "we really work well as a team."

This objective of member relationship maintenance or strengthening seems apparent enough, but it does not receive the amount of recognition that the objective of goal achievement does, frequently it is not trained for, and occasionally, it is not even allowed to be discussed. However, a group of people cannot function truly as a team without both components being addressed.

WHO MAKES A TEAM?

If one uses the definition of a team as two or more people who work together, then anyone is a team member, even if it is for a one-day period. However, using Gillies' criteria, one can divide the "who's" into two distinct groupings: (1) the official or nucleus members and (2) the unofficial members. Official members are those who participate in both objectives of goal achievement and relationship maintenance. Using the pediatric nephrology team at St. Louis Children's Hospital as an example, the official team members are:

- the patient and family members
- the attending level nephrologists
- the fellows in nephrology training
- the renal clinical nurse specialist
- the renal social worker
- the renal dietitian
- the patient care manager of the patient unit
- the secretary
- the patient care manager of the dialysis unit
- the dialysis nursing staff and the school teacher

An attempt is made to incorporate any rotating residents or medical students into this team when they are electively assigned to the nephrology service. Frequently the chaplain will move in and out of this team network.

The specifics of how these members function and interrelate will be looked at shortly, but generally, one could say they function and behave much like a family—a social system that can be analyzed by systems theory. The unofficial members are individuals who "work" with this team but by definition are primarily functioning and behaving for only one objective: the achievement of some specific goal or task. Such unofficial team members might be:

- staff nurses
- outpatient personnel
- Visiting Nurses Association (VNA) or other agencies; schools
- hospital department individuals
- transplant team members
- private physicians
- students
- medical house officers
- consulting teams

Often one belongs to more than one team; for example, the pediatric renal clinical nurse specialist belongs to the renal team, the clinical specialist team, and the nursing staff team on the patient care unit for renal patients.

All future references to team members in this chapter will be of official team members only.

CHARACTERISTICS OF INDIVIDUAL TEAM MEMBERS

Team members bring with them a host of characteristics, values, perceptions, assumptions, and skills that greatly influence how they behave both in task achievement activities as well as in relationship activities. The following generalizations are meant only as possible considerations of how individuals might behave; these characteristics may or may not hold true. They are referred to here only to begin an analysis of the numerous influencing factors in team functioning.

Physicians

By and large, physicians are achievement oriented, motivated, dedicated, accountable, and dominant individuals. Generally, they view themselves as "captains of the ship," the leaders in charge.[16] They perceive that the patient and the care for that patient are their responsibility. "Physicians make decisions on nursing, diet, etc. and yet have no training in these areas."[17] Frequently, due to this strong commitment to leadership, they are unaccustomed to seeking consult or counsel from others.[18] Chaska even states that physicians are taught that sharing means abandonment.[19] Their medical orientation tends to direct them toward long-term outcomes (rather than eight-hour work periods) being mostly task oriented toward health issues restrictively. The definitions and limitations inflicted by law are ever present in their decision making. Their realistic valuing of nursing or other professions is frequently limited, but it often is influenced by their inability to see the need to understand it. The perception that nursing is helpful as a second profession to medicine is not an uncommon one.[20] Lee concluded from her study that "of the few physicians who do recognize nursing as having its own standards, skills, procedures, and body of knowledge, virtually none can conceive of nursing care as something distinct from medical care, though they acknowledge that it does have something extra to offer."[21]

And, of course, the majority of physicians are males. (See Chapter 5 for additional references to this topic.)

Nurses

The majority of nurses are females, and so the women's movement has been influential. By and large, nurses are more passive, more motherly, and have a stronger need to please and nurture.[22] Their professional image is usually viewed as less important than that of physicians by themselves and others.[23] Often, defensive behaviors are based on this status difference.[24] Nurses frequently view their relationships with physicians as beyond their control.[25] Open disagreement is to be avoided, and "failure to play the games was seen by nurses to result in immediate loss in communication, inability to establish a working relationship with the doctor, ostracism, and frequent elimination," as reported in a study conducted by DeYoung.[26] Nurses appear to have two separate standards for themselves: to think and make self-decisions and to please and follow others' decisions. These two are in conflict and are incompatible with each other, and frequently the passive role wins out.[27]

One finds it unusual for a nurse, even if skilled, to supervise a physician in any kind of situation.[28] Some nurses do model their roles on the functions of physicians, taking refuge, however, in the legal definitions and limitations of nursing.[29] Morgan discussed the nurse "game" of sharing in medical practice without seeming to do so.[30] This can set the stage for less accountability and decreased responsibility on the whole, as frequently seen by nurses who feel that what occurs to patients after their shift is over is not of concern to them. Nursing, in general, is oriented more to the patient directly, but is directed by preset, scheduled nursing activities that are task oriented. Most objectives of nurses' behaviors, as well as those for the patients, are defined in shorter timeframes—a more "here and now" orientation.[31] Regardless, more nursing time is spent with patients than is physician time. (See Chapter 5 for further information.)

Social Workers, Dietitians, Physical Therapists, Pharmacists

These professional groups are also primarily made up of females. The priorities for patients from their individual perspectives is often very different from that of nursing or medicine—not necessarily in conflict, just different. Their ability to understand nursing and medicine is limited in spite of what might be a close working relationship, and vice versa. There is not a great deal in the literature regarding the relationships of these and other professionals with physicians or nurses.

Clients/Patients

Often this group of persons is not included as team members. Patients frequently perceive the physician as leader. They have perceptions of nursing and other professionals that will influence the roles and relationships that result. Clients/patients are frequently fearful of voicing their opinions or of not taking charge in any way, with resultant feelings of passivity and inability to participate or control their lives. Health care is viewed differently by the public than other purchased services, and behaviors are therefore different. For example, one frequently hears "what did he or she say?" when a health professional leaves the room. In a department store, the client would generally ask directly if information was not understood.

Each group of members on any given team frequently has a different orientation and priority and is limited in the understanding of the others. Often one group is not privy to others' decision-making rationale, which is often dehumanizing and frustrating.[32]

TOTAL TEAM INTERRELATIONSHIPS

Space has been given in this chapter, as well as in the literature reviewed, to relationships among individuals. Obviously, this is important since many day-to-day activities and decisions are based on such relationships. However, there is another important piece to team functioning, and that is the collective relationship of the team. This, like individual relationships, is a part of the "maintenance or strengthening" component and does not need to be left to chance. As Chaska states, a team must spend time working on its own functioning process—treating itself as a patient, periodically diagnosing its own state of health.[33]

Many teams function almost exclusively from various one-to-one relationships, seldom coming together as a collective group. This in itself is a barrier to true team functioning. Other teams do have total group interactions, but the dynamics of such are seldom evaluated for effectiveness.

As with any system or family, the whole is often different and greater than the sum of the parts.

RELEVANT FACTORS IN TOTAL GROUP INTERACTION

The interaction of the total group needs to be viewed as a social setting with specific functioning ground rules. The understanding of these rules, as well as the resultant behaviors and consequences, can lead to alterations in barriers or growth of positive elements in order to foster team development and functioning. "Failure to address the relationship itself leaves the development of good relationships to chance."[34]

Purposes

What theme or themes has brought this total group together? Are the objectives primarily social, work, or educational? Is the theme the same each time? How clearly are these themes or purposes understood by the members? Do these interactions occur on a regularly scheduled basis or are they "called" by certain members for specific reasons?

Questions such as these can be helpful in two ways. First, they can identify a frequent area of discord for some team members who perceive the purpose of a total group meeting to be different from other members' perceptions. Second, they might help to identify a means to increase the outcome potential of team interactions. Obviously, the identification of the objectives of any group gathering or interaction determines the time and agenda required.

Setting

What setting factors exist that can be used to help identify what processes are occurring? What type of location is generally selected? Is the same setting used each time? What type of seating arrangement does the team usually end up using? Does the setting fit the purpose of the team meeting?

Does the institution encourage group meetings by providing time, space, and equipment? What is the size of the group, and how does this influence interactions? How formal or sophisticated are the interactions? Is humor allowed? What environmental influences are accepted? Do people come and go; are a lot of interruptions tolerated? Do people show up on time or not show up at all? What is the true frequency of such gatherings?

Frequently the inappropriate selection of the setting creates a major barrier to the accomplishment of the objectives a team desires. For example, team rounds conducted at the patient bedside often preclude the ability to add the component of socialization and interpersonal sharing among team members. Group gatherings during the busiest part of the day often lead to interruptions and the inability to foster the educational component. The crowdedness as well as the ability to visualize all members present greatly influence human behaviors.

Roles

What roles do people play? Gillies identifies some usual roles common to groups: the idea generators, the evaluators, the problem solvers, and the moral supporters.[35] Are these or other roles recognized by the other team members? Are these people trained in any way for these roles? Do certain people function in the same role consistently, or do they rotate roles depending on certain factors? Are there real leaders in the group? How many leaders are there? Is there competition for leadership? Do different people lead under different circumstances or regarding different issues? Is the leadership style one of an autocratic or democratic nature? Is there a social power to the role of leader and therefore carried by only selective members? Is this social power used to impel others to act in certain ways? Is leadership or power attributed to given persons by the other members? If so, is it done directly or indirectly? Do sex roles determine role selections? Are there followers? Are there facilitators or saboteurs? What value is given to these roles? Is there a hierarchy to the group, and if so, what kind of hierarchy?

The issue of roles and group dynamics is a complex one and cannot be addressed adequately in a brief section. These questions can, however, begin a process of evaluation for the purpose of learning a few valuable points about any group interactions. The process of change can never be accomplished without this first step. Team interactions can be evaluated by use of systems theory, which recognizes the need for reciprocal interactions of individuals: one cannot have leaders without followers, nor equality in the face of hierarchy. The dynamics of any group are anything but static, which require close assessment: an alteration in the roles and functions of anyone within the system will bring about change in all others as well as in the system itself.[36]

Communication

What is the communication style of the group? Is it "closed" or "open"?[37] What are the effects of, the effectiveness of, and the satisfaction resulting from the communication patterns used. Often communication patterns in a group differ from the usual communication patterns occurring among given individuals because of the very condition of being observed by others.[38] What effects does this have, and in what way does the communication pattern change?

Close assessment of communication patterns often reveals poor listening skills, assumption making, defensiveness, or manipulations. All communication among humans carries both a direct and indirect component, which are of equal importance. Are these two components in agreement or contradiction: for example, do people ask a question in the form of a demand or make factual statements when really asking a question? Is the underlying premise that others should be able to "read minds"?

Change

Are the interactions of the group predictable?[39] What developmental stages has the group undergone over time? What phases of change does it go through regularly? What happens when some member is absent or a temporary new member enters the group? How easy is it for new members to join? How difficult is it to rid the group of "misfits"? Why do people join the group? Do all team members have a say in who joins the group? What systems are used to problem solve?

Again, systems theory or change theory can provide useful means by which to evaluate this important component of team interactions. The incorporation of new team members into an already functioning team is often a stressful time and frequently not planned for or discussed openly. The temporary or permanent loss of a key role member is likewise relevant.

Togetherness

What values does the group hold most precious? What value does the group give members for their usefulness to the group as a whole? Is there a sense of wholeness or togetherness? What expectations, insecurities, rewards, or threats exist? How are differences dealt with? Do members understand the differences that exist regarding other members' professional roles? Is there a personal support system? How is assistance asked for and given? What rescuing patterns occur? What are the group's comradeship characteristics? What is the level of self-awareness skills of individual members? What is the capability of mutual influence? What elements of dependence, independence, and interdependence exist? What is the ratio of professional representation?

Gillies notes that some of the characteristics of togetherness are (1) that each group has its own characteristic behaviors, habits, and flavor despite replacement of individuals, (2) that each group tends to respond as a whole to stimuli directed at its parts, and (3) that strong pressure is exerted toward uniformity of behavior and attitude.[40] One generally notes a shared value system among members of such a group. There is a sense of caring and concern for individual members. A comfortableness exists that fosters growth and problem solving.

Much like in a family, a sense of belonging often compels individuals to join a team. Occasionally persons strive to become team members, feeling that belonging to a group of professionals with perceived higher status will bring them the same. Frequently this motive results in frustration and a sense of dependency.

Chaska discusses the expectations of most team members: (1) that they deliver the best care they know how, (2) that they maintain credibility of expertise, and (3) that they be protected from limitations on effective practice that are arbitrary and serve no necessary purpose.[41] Are these expectations of others communicated directly or indirectly?

Interestingly, as defined previously, the patient and families are often viewed as official team members and can fit into this theme of "togetherness" even if not physically present at many team gatherings. More than likely, all team members will represent various factors and serve as liaisons. Such is often true with nursing representation on any given team; a single nurse might indeed represent a whole nursing staff, giving the team a sense of extended "togetherness."

Occasionally one sees confusion between the "togetherness" concept and a "must agree" syndrome. All individual team members should and will bring with them a variety of values, perceptions, skills, and opinions. This will obviously lead to differences. Togetherness represents only a valuing of the process to arrive at a mutually agreeable solution.

Tasks/Activities

How are tasks delegated or distributed? What skills do individual team members have? How flexible or rigid is the system in changing tasks? What evaluation system occurs (internal or external) regarding outcome of task effectiveness? What reward or punishment system exists? What tasks hold the highest value by the group? How does reassignment of tasks occur when team members are absent?

Wilson looks at the influence of one profession on the tasks and activities of others and how, if not mutually agreed upon, conflict can occur. For example, the decision by the medical staff to "No Code" a patient can and will influence the tasks and activities of the nursing staff.[42] Chaska discusses this issue of tasks, stating that if the task at hand requires very specialized skills, generally there is very little conflict.[43] However, conflict can arise when specialization or skill does not determine task assignment or when individuals fail to recognize that it is not the task itself that is in question but the interpersonal relationship process involved in task delegation. Chaska suggests that assignment be made on the basis of (1) time availability, (2) liking of task, (3) cost, (4) number of people available, (5) supply and demand requirements, (6) seniority or status, (7) focus of care, and (8) nature of requirements for care.[44]

AWARENESS OF OBJECTIVE OF "TEAM MAINTENANCE" AS AN IMPORTANT FUNCTION

"Failure to address the relationship itself leaves the development of good relationships to chance."[45] Since this quote has been used two or three times it is not only important but is the major problem with poorly functioning teams. But how does one go about taking charge of incorporating this important component into every day (and ongoing) team functioning? First, one or more persons on the team need to take the responsibility for such. Initially, reading and learning more about group and systems theory might be very beneficial. Then there should be a period of concrete observation to evaluate team interactions, strengths, weaknesses, barriers, and resources that truly exist.

Due to my personal interests in interpersonal relationships, I took on this role many years ago with the renal team with which I was working. The addition of a social worker to our team added a valuable resource as well as adding perspective and skill to the ongoing evaluation process of our team's interactions. Since then, almost *all* of the team members have recognized and begun to value and work toward this major component of team functioning.

Alterations in Communication Patterns

Frequently, assessments of group communication patterns indicate the use of indirect styles; hints and clues to the true nature of the communication are sent by non-verbal pathways rather than stated directly in words. Misinterpretation of the clues or feelings of manipulation can result from indirect communications.

The establishment of direct communication patterns can begin with any individual taking the responsibility for saying exactly what one means when talking with any other individual or with the group. Stopping and asking oneself, "What exactly do I wish to say?" then sending the entire message in words, and lastly, asking the receiver(s) if the message was clearly perceived are all important steps in direct communications. The use of paraphrasing ("What I think you are saying is. . . .") or asking for clarification ("I'm not sure I understand what you mean by. . . .") are extremely useful in attempting to be sure one has clearly perceived another individual's communications.

After a team interaction has occurred where goals or tasks have been discussed, it is beneficial for one member to take the responsibility to summarize by asking, "Okay, now exactly what is it we are all trying to accomplish here?" or "If I understand correctly, we have decided that I am going to do . . ., and you are going to do. . . ."

A vital component to effective communication is to immediately seek clarification of messages that the receiver perceives in a way that results in a highly charged emotional state. I would like to share an example that addresses this type of situation. A new physician had recently joined our team in a training fellowship. Part of his orientation did include an orientation to the role of clinical nurse specialist both by myself and other team members. One day while working in a busy clinic, Dr. X had just completed his examination of the patient, and I went into the room to continue an ongoing education program with the child and family. Dr. X was overheard to say that there were other patients he could see if the room I was occupying were vacant. I found myself to be angry, perceiving his message to mean his team contribution was more valuable than mine.

This situation and others like it give one several options: do nothing, *indirectly* communicate back to the sender one's disapproval, or *directly* communicate to the sender your perceptions and ask for clarification to the true meaning of the message. Upon choosing the latter, I approached Dr. X, stating that I may have misinterpreted his message and wished not to do so. He admitted that he perceived that I was "socializing" with the patient and felt that not to be of value during a busy clinic. Discussion of the goals for this child and family followed, which helped to clarify the functions of the clinical specialist. Dr. X then asked that I include him in subsequent teaching sessions so he might learn more about the educational programs our team provides for our patients.

SETTING THE STAGE FOR MUTUAL DECISION MAKING

Often mutual decision making does occur within teams, but it is restricted to random one-to-one interactions that only a few team members may be faced with at some point in time. Even more frequently, however, mutual decision making does not occur at all: unilateral decisions are made by a physician regarding medical care or by a nurse regarding nursing care. Both are less than optimal.

The benefits of mutual decision making regarding health care delivery have been discussed previously in this chapter. Each team needs to assess exactly which components of patient care require mutual input. Because this issue is usually not *directly* discussed, the potential for conflict surfaces. A total team gathering to outline the areas of mutuality is essential. Team members need to communicate clearly to their fellow team members in what areas they wish to be included and how *much* input they wish to have. Often team members will only wish to be knowledgeable of the decisions others are making versus being an integral part of the decision-making process.

The main avenue for mutual decision making with the team at St. Louis Children's Hospital occurs through "renal rounds." Such rounds were a routine part of the team's activities when I first joined the team. The purposes of these rounds (understood well by all) were (1) to discuss the medical problems of all inhouse patients, (2) to provide a teaching forum, since our facility is a teaching and training institution, and (3) to provide some social interaction time for the team members. All physicians were encouraged to attend these rounds, and the setting was one of openness for suggestions and problem solving of the medical situations the team was encountering. Rarely did nurses, social workers, or other professionals attend. These rounds were held Wednesday evenings and Saturday mornings and frequently lasted a couple of hours.

Upon my initial assessment of the team functions and interactions, it was apparent that the medical members of this team indeed were making mutual decisions regarding the medical care of the renal patients. The unity and likeness in treatment plans often stemmed from group discussions and learning. Alterations in treatment or new treatment programs were always a result of group discussions.

This seemed like the perfect format to begin to include other professions into the overall teamwork. I began attending these rounds on a regular basis. Soon it became apparent that the Saturday rounds were generally more hurried in nature and did not seem as conducive to the addition of other information for discussion. I benefited tremendously by attending the Wednesday rounds, learning the rationale for medical decisions. The team was very accepting of my requests for explanations if I was unclear. My presence soon became normal, and the opportunity arose for me to introduce other subject matter to the usual discussions. Teaching programs soon developed, and my ability to add relevant nursing, psychosocial, developmental, or interrelationship issues to the overall planning was forthcoming. Soon the physicians began to see and hear the benefits of the expanded outcomes, which encouraged my visibility even more. The addition of our social worker to the team meant that she, too, began to come to rounds, which broadened our planning and implementation skills even further. Now the patient care managers of the patient units, as well as the renal dietitian, attend regularly. Staff nurses are invited but find it difficult to take the extended time to attend. Often a primary nurse will attend if some critical issue is going to be discussed. Generally speaking, however, I and the patient care managers serve as the interteam links to facilitate the passing of information to the primary nurse or to give input to the team regarding some new and important information that the primary nurse has gained.

A second format for mutual giving and sharing of information for the purpose of mutual decision making is the use of joint record keeping. St. Louis Children's Hospital has for years utilized joint progress recordings, which has allowed other disciplines to offer information to the overall team.

The concept of risk-taking in sharing is relevant to this discussion. I can well remember the insecurities and even fears in asking questions, offering suggestions, and voicing my opinions. Obviously, the manner in which this is done is vital. I agree with previously noted authors that it felt risky, and there was fear that mistakes would bring large consequences.[46] Respecting my own knowledge and skills had to come before such respect could be expected from my fellow team members. Blackwood addresses this issue by saying that "we can't suddenly rush out and demand the equal recognition and equal say with physicians as if others owe that to us."[47] Nurses, like all other professionals represented on a team, must communicate their input in a manner that maximizes receptiveness by other professionals, but as discussed earlier, they must not assume that such input will be understood or accepted readily, since other professionals frequently are educated and trained to think in terms of other priorities. Keeping the perspective of complementary rather than competitive roles and input is essential.

Mutuality can extend beyond just decision making within teams. The equal use of titles fosters mutual level communications. Frequently nurses refer to physicians by their professional name while physicians call nurses by their first name. Mauksch addresses this issue and offers suggestions for alterations.[48] Likewise, making oneself available for socialization opportunities with other members of the team can do a lot to change socially stereotyped roles and behaviors and enhance the humanization component of interrelationships. Asking a physician or the social worker to join you for lunch or coffee demonstrates a willingness to relate to them in areas other than health and patient care. Centrally located office or working areas allow the visibility of various team members, which can be extremely beneficial.

ALTERING DEFENSIVE BEHAVIORS

Defensive behaviors serve no constructive purpose whatsoever, but they are easily aroused and easily perpetuated in our present system and society as a whole. Many of the factors contributing to this arena have been alluded to earlier and in other chapters. Mauksch suggests that informality and openness work well to replace formality and deviousness.[49] I would add that risk taking is also necessary—risk taking in doing what one feels one can do in any given situation without holding back out of fear or anger. Mauksch discusses how many nurses feel a real anger because they are not asked their opinions or for their input.[50] My response to that is, have they ever asked to be asked—I mean directly asked to be asked? Or have they ever offered (appropriately) to demonstrate that they indeed have something to offer? This author strongly agrees with Rodgers' statement that arguments or discord are usually more symbolic (the emotional component) than substantive (the factual component).[51] I well remember times when I offered an opinion or a piece of information and it was not accepted. I can remember allowing myself to have feelings of rejection or disapproval. Then I became aware that these same team members challenged the opinions even of their own professional group—so that was the norm, not the exception. I then followed the norm that was used in those situations: either verifying my statements with facts or theories or asking the group to allow me to test my assumptions and return to them with the outcome. I certainly recognize that I prefer not to have someone demand that I follow a certain decision, so my attempts to demand would be inappropriate also.

Winker discusses some do's and don'ts that are useful: (1) respect each individual for his or her contributions, (2) focus on common goals, (3) be comfortable in one's own role, (4) be aware of one's own role, (5) speak from one's own professional knowledge, (6) don't function from a "bottle" frame of mind, (7) take care regarding vindictiveness, (8) don't try to take over other professionals' roles, (9) don't try to take on characteristics of other professionals, and (10) don't try to offer "superior" advice on someone else's professional knowledge base.[52]

Self-confidence plays a vital part in the equation of team relationships. The state of emotional defensiveness that results from falling victim to the dependence traps (of maintaining one's self-esteem and self-confidence only through the eyes of others) must be avoided. Phillips discusses this issue and says nurses frequently feel dissatisfaction because physicians do not give recognition to services rendered.[53] The illogical premise here is that nurses are rendering services to physicians. The line between working "with" someone and working "for" someone can be very thin sometimes. However, the resulting emotional states can be very different.

To move toward interdependency in a team relationship, individual members must recognize themselves for what they are and take full responsibility for their own functioning and feelings of self-worth. One must have an already established secure sense of professional identity. Then and only then can one open oneself to review and appraisal from professional colleagues in other professions.[54]

OTHER FACILITATORS

The concept of primary nursing is the closest mode of delivering nursing care in a truly team manner (not to be interpreted as "team nursing"). Individuals work on a continuous basis with the same professionals involved from beginning to discharge. The continuity then sets the stage for the component of relationship maintenance or strengthening to occur, or at least to become visible.

The concept of family centered care incorporates the patient and family into the team by expanding the focus of health care beyond the delivery of medical care objectives and as a result requires a variety of other professional groups to become necessary resources.

Also, the philosophies of the administrative directors of any given institution do much to facilitate or hinder team activities. The policies and communication channels established frequently determine individuals' abilities to function independently in small team activities.

EDUCATION

A long-term suggestion that could indeed facilitate the accomplishment of good team functioning is that of incorporating team interaction into the curricula of all health care professional training programs. Some programs might offer this in a theoretical manner, but few have practical experiences for using the concept.[55,56] One such program was discussed in the literature where the sole purpose of a semester of clinical experience for both medical and nursing students was to learn about the other professional roles to gain relationship experience in the day-to-day routine of delivering patient care.[57]

SUMMARY

A team is something more than people working together. The concept of the team carries two vital components—the "what" they do and "how" they do it together. Each individual brings important personal and professional qualities. However, group dynamics and interactions are issues of equal importance.

This chapter offers suggestions not only on how to look at the above factors, but to overcome barriers and facilitate the development of true team functioning.

NOTES

1. Norma L. Chaska, *The Nursing Profession: Views Through the Mist* (New York: McGraw-Hill Book Company, 1978), p. 325.

2. Margaret L. Pluckhan, "A Problem Affecting the Delivery of Health Care," *Nursing Forum* 9, no. 3 (1972): 310.

3. Cynthia K. Winker and Nancy C. Lee, "Developing a Joint Practice Team," *Dimensions of Critical Care Nursing* 1, no. 6 (November–December 1982): 363.

4. Margaret L. Pluckhan, "A Problem Affecting the Delivery of Health Care," *Nursing Forum* 9, no. 3 (1972): 304.

5. Ingeborg G. Mauksch and Michael H. Miller, *Implementing Change in Nursing* (St. Louis, Mo.: C.V. Mosby Co., 1981), p. 84.

6. Dee Ann Gillies, *Nursing Management: A Systems Approach* (Philadelphia: W.B. Saunders Co., 1982), p. 158.

7. T. Audean Duespohl, *Nursing in Transition* (Rockville, Md.: Aspen Systems Corporation, 1983), p. 237.

8. Pamela McNutt Devereux, "Nurse/Physician Collaboration: Nursing Practice Considerations," *The Journal of Nursing Administration*, September 1981, p. 38.

9. Gloria Jo Floyd and Billy Don Smith, "Job Enrichment," *Nursing Management* 14, no. 5 (May 1983): 22.

10. Timothy Sheard, "The Structure of Conflict in Nurse Physician Relations," *Supervisor Nurse*, August 1980, p. 14.

11. Pamela McNutt Devereux, "Nurse/Physician Collaboration: Nursing Practice Considerations," *The Journal of Nursing Administration*, September 1981, p. 38.

12. Carol D. DeYoung, Margene Tower, and Jody Glittenburg, *Out of Uniform and Into Trouble, Again: The Nurse's Role in Community Mental Health Centers and Other Places* (Thorofare, N.J.: Slack, Inc., 1971), p. 23.

13. Dee Ann Gillies, *Nursing Management: A Systems Approach* (Philadelphia: W.B. Saunders Co., 1982), p. 150.

14. Ibid.

15. Ibid.

16. Ingeborg G. Mauksch and Michael H. Miller, *Implementing Change in Nursing* (St. Louis, Mo.: C.V. Mosby Co., 1981), p. 74.

17. Ibid.

18. T. Audean Duespohl, *Nursing in Transition* (Rockville, Md.: Aspen Systems Corporation, 1983), p. 237.

19. Norma L. Chaska, *The Nursing Profession: Views Through the Mist* (New York: McGraw-Hill Book Company, 1978), p. 338.

20. Carol D. DeYoung, Margene Tower, and Jody Glittenburg, *Out of Uniform and Into Trouble, Again: The Nurse's Role in Community Mental Health Centers and Other Places* (Thorofare, N.J.: Slack, Inc., 1971), p. 25.

21. Anthony A. Lee, "How Nurses Rate with M.D.'s: Still the Handmaiden," *RN,* July 1979, p. 21.

22. Carol D. DeYoung, Margene Tower, and Jody Glittenburg, *Out of Uniform and Into Trouble, Again: The Nurse's Role in Community Mental Health Centers and Other Places* (Thorofare, N.J.: Slack, Inc., 1971), p. 29.

23. Ingeborg G. Mauksch and Michael H. Miller, *Implementing Change in Nursing* (St. Louis, Mo.: C.V. Mosby Co., 1981), p. 85.

24. Carol D. DeYoung, Margene Tower, and Jody Glittenburg, *Out of Uniform and Into Trouble, Again: The Nurse's Role in Community Mental Health Centers and Other Places* (Thorofare, N.J.: Slack, Inc., 1971), p. 24.

25. Cynthia K. Winker and Nancy C. Lee, "Developing a Joint Practice Team," *Dimensions of Critical Care Nursing* 1, no. 6 (November–December 1982): 360.

26. Carol D. DeYoung, Margene Tower, and Jody Glittenburg, *Out of Uniform and Into Trouble, Again: The Nurse's Role in Community Mental Health Centers and Other Places* (Thorofare, N.J.: Slack, Inc., 1971), p. 26.

27. Charles K. Hofling et al., "An Experimental Study in Nurse-Physician Relationships," *The Journal of Nervous and Mental Disease* 143, no. 2 (1966): 179.

28. Carol D. DeYoung, Margene Tower, and Jody Glittenburg, *Out of Uniform and Into Trouble, Again: The Nurse's Role in Community Mental Health Centers and Other Places* (Thorofare, N.J.: Slack, Inc., 1971), p. 32.

29. Pamela McNutt Devereux, "Nurse/Physician Collaboration: Nursing Practice Considerations," *The Journal of Nursing Administration,* September 1981, p. 37.

30. Ann P. Morgan and Janice M. McCann, "Nurse-Physician Relationships: The Ongoing Conflict," *Nursing Administration Quarterly,* Summer 1983, p. 4.

31. Ingeborg G. Mauksch and Michael H. Miller, *Implementing Change in Nursing* (St. Louis, Mo.: C.V. Mosby Co., 1981), p. 74.

32. T. Audean Duespohl, *Nursing in Transition* (Rockville, Md.: Aspen Systems Corporation, 1983), p. 234.

33. Norma L. Chaska, *The Nursing Profession: Views Through the Mist* (New York: McGraw-Hill Book Company, 1978), p. 340.

34. Pamela McNutt Devereux, "Nurse/Physician Collaboration: Nursing Practice Considerations," *The Journal of Nursing Administration,* September 1981, p. 38.

35. Dee Ann Gillies, *Nursing Management: A Systems Approach* (Philadelphia: W.B. Saunders Co., 1982), p. 153.

36. John R. Phillips, "Health Care Provides Relationships: A Matter of Reciprocity," *Nursing Outlook,* November 1979, p. 738.

37. Ann Marriner, *The Nursing Process: A Scientific Approach to Nursing Care* (St. Louis, Mo.: C.V. Mosby Co., 1975).

38. Dee Ann Gillies, *Nursing Management: A Systems Approach* (Philadelphia: W.B. Saunders Co., 1982), p. 151.

39. Ann Marriner, *The Nursing Process: A Scientific Approach to Nursing Care* (St. Louis, Mo.: C.V. Mosby Co., 1975).

40. Dee Ann Gillies, *Nursing Management: A Systems Approach* (Philadelphia: W.B. Saunders Co., 1982), p. 152.

41. Norma L. Chaska, *The Nursing Profession: Views Through the Mist* (New York: McGraw-Hill Book Company, 1978), p. 345.

42. Jane Wilson, "Ethics and the Physician-Nurse Relationship," *Canadian Medical Association Journal* 129 (August 1, 1983): 290.

43. Norma L. Chaska, *The Nursing Profession: Views Through the Mist* (New York: McGraw-Hill Book Company, 1978), p. 325.

44. Norma L. Chaska, *The Nursing Profession: Views Through the Mist* (New York: McGraw-Hill Book Company, 1978), p. 325.

45. Pamela McNutt Devereux, "Nurse/Physician Collaboration: Nursing Practice Considerations," *The Journal of Nursing Administration*, September 1981, p. 38.

46. Carol D. DeYoung, Margene Tower, and Jody Glittenburg, *Out of Uniform and Into Trouble, Again: The Nurse's Role in Community Mental Health Centers and Other Places* (Thorofare, N.J.: Slack, Inc., 1971), p. 23.

47. Sarah A. Blackwood, "At This Hospital, 'The Captain of the Ship' is Dead," *RN*, March 1979, p. 94.

48. Ingeborg G. Mauksch and Michael H. Miller, *Implementing Change in Nursing* (St. Louis, Mo.: C.V. Mosby Co., 1981), pp. 74–76.

49. Ibid., p. 84.

50. Ibid.

51. Janet A. Rodgers, "For Nursing or Against Medicine: A Group Replay of the Second Individual Process," *Nursing Outlook*, August 1981, p. 480.

52. Cynthia K. Winker and Nancy C. Lee, "Developing a Joint Practice Team," *Dimensions of Critical Care Nursing* 1, no. 6 (November–December 1982): 363.

53. John R. Phillips, "Health Care Provides Relationships: A Matter of Reciprocity," *Nursing Outlook*, November 1979, p. 740.

54. Janet A. Rodgers, "For Nursing or Against Medicine: A Group Replay of the Second Individual Process," *Nursing Outlook*, August 1981, p. 480.

55. Norma L. Chaska, *The Nursing Profession: Views Through the Mist* (New York: McGraw-Hill Book Company, 1978), p. 333.

56. Pamela McNutt Devereux, "Nurse/Physician Collaboration: Nursing Practice Considerations," *The Journal of Nursing Administration*, September 1981, pp. 37–39.

57. Ibid.

SUGGESTED READINGS

Altschul, A. "With All Due Respect . . . Interprofessional Relations." *Nursing Mirror* 157, no. 2 (1983): 20.

American Nurses Association. *Nursing—A Social Policy Statement.* Kansas City, Mo.: ANA, 1980.

Blackwood, Sarah A. "At This Hospital, 'The Captain of the Ship' is Dead." *RN*, March 1979, pp. 77–94.

Chaska, Norma L., ed. *The Nursing Profession: Views Through the Mist.* New York: McGraw-Hill Book Company, 1978.

Chaska, Norma L. *The Nursing Profession: A Time to Speak.* New York: McGraw-Hill Book Company, 1983.

Devereux, Pamela M. "Essential Elements of Nurse-Physician Collaboration." *Journal of Nursing Administration* 5 (May 11, 1981): 19–23.

Devereux, Pamela M. "Nurse/Physician Collaboration: Nursing Practice Considerations." *Journal of Nursing Administration,* September 1981, pp. 37–39.

DeYoung, Carol; Tower, Margene; and Glittenburg, Jody. *Out of Uniform and Into Trouble, Again: The Nurse's Role in Community Mental Health Centers and Other Places.* Thorofare, N.J.: Slack, Inc., 1971, pp. 22–34.

"Doctors, Nurses Must Discuss Differences, Work Together." *Hospitals* 52, no. 24 (December 16, 1978): 17–18.

Dopson, L. "Lines of Communication." *Nursing Times* 75, no. 14 (April 5, 1979): 567.

Duespohl, T.A. *Nursing in Transition.* Rockville, Md: Aspen Systems Corp., 1983.

Erde, E.L. "Notions of Teams and Team Talk in Health Care: Implications for Responsibilities." *Law-Med-Health-Care* 9, no. 5 (October 1981): 26–28.

Floyd, Gloria Jo, and Smith, Billy Don. "Job Enrichment." *Nursing Management* 14, no. 5 (May 1983): 22.

Friedman, F.B. "A Nurse's Guide to the Care and Handling of M.D.s." *RN* 45, no. 3 (March 1982): 39–43, 118–120.

Furnham, A.; Pendleton, D.; and Manicom, C. "The Perception of Different Occupations Within the Medical Profession." *Soc-Sci-Med (E)* 15, no. 4 (November 1981): 289–300.

Gillies, Dee Ann. *Nursing Management: A Systems Approach.* Philadelphia: W.B. Saunders, 1982, pp. 150–159.

Giovinco, G. "Interpersonal/Professional Relationship: Some Critical Issues Involving the Nurse, the Physician and the Patient." *Journal of Nursing Ethics* 1, no. 1 (Fall 1978): 13–16.

Glen, S. "Stop Pandering to Doctors." *Nursing Mirror* 154, no. 25 (June 23, 1982): 48–49.

Grubb, L.L. "Nurse-Physician Collaboration." *Supervisor Nurse* 10, no. 3 (March 1979): 16–21.

Hirata, I., Jr. "Togetherness—The Health Care Team." *Journal of the American College Health Association* 29, no. 1 (August 1980): 5–6.

Hofling, Charles K. et al., "An Experimental Study in Nurse-Physician Relationships." *The Journal of Mental and Nervous Disease* 143, no. 2: 171–180.

Johnston, P.F. "Improving the Nurse-Physician Relationship." *Journal of Nursing Administration* 13, no. 3 (March 1983): 19–20.

Lang, D.A., and Goertzen, I. "Doctors vs Nurses: Is Anybody Winning?" *Nursing Careers* 2, no. 4 (September–October 1981): 16–17.

Larson, Magali Sarfatti. *The Rise of Professionalism—A Sociological Analysis.* Los Angeles: University of California Press, 1977.

Lee, A.A. "How Nurses Rate with M.D.'s: Still the Handmaiden." *RN* 42, no. 7 (July 1979): 20–30.

Lynch, B.L. "Team Building: Will It Work in Health Care?" *Journal of Allied Health* 10, no. 4 (November 1981): 240–247.

Marriner, Ann. *The Nursing Process: A Scientific Approach to Nursing Care.* St. Louis, Mo.: C.V. Mosby Co., 1975.

Martin, J.C. "Hospital Problems Need Interprofessional Approach." *Dimensions of Health Service* 56, no. 8 (August 1979): 8–9.

Mauksch, Ingeborg G., and Miller, Michael H. *Implementing Change in Nursing.* St. Louis, Mo.: C.V. Mosby Co., 1981, pp. 73–86.

Mausch, Ingeborg G. "Nurse-physician Collaboration: A Changing Relationship." *Journal of Nursing Administration* 11, no. 6 (June 1981): 35–38.

McGuire, M.A. "Nurse-physician Interactions: Silence Isn't Golden." *Supervisor Nurse* 11, no. 3 (March 11, 1980): 36–39.

Morgan, A.P., and McCann, J.M. "Nurse-physician Relationships: The Ongoing Conflict." *Nursing Administration Quarterly* 7, no. 4 (Summer 1983): 1–7.

Murphy, L.M. "War Lords One, Nurses Zero." *RN* 41, no. 10 (October 1978): 45–46.

Pawsat, E.H. "The New Horizon Nurse and the Physician: A Need for Guidelines." *Wisconsin Medical Journal* 80, no. 11 (November 1981): 15–17.

Phillips, J.R. "Health Care Provider Relationships a Matter of Reciprocity." *Nursing Outlook* 27, no. 11 (November 1979): 738–741.

Pluckhan, Margaret L. "Professional Territoriality: A Problem Affecting the Delivery of Health Care." *Nursing Forum* 11, no. 3 (1972): 300–310.

Ride, T. "Do We Understand the Process?" *Nursing Mirror* 157, no. 7 (August 17, 1983): 12–13.

Ritter, H.A. "Nurse-physician Collaboration." *Connecticut Medical Journal* 45, no. 1 (January 1981): 23–25.

Rodgers, J.A. "Toward Professional Adulthood." *Nursing Outlook* 29, no. 8 (August 1981): 478–481.

Schreckenberger, Paul C. "Playing for the Health Team." *Journal of the American Medical Association* 213, no. 2 (July 30, 1970): 279–281.

Schwartzbaum, A.; McGrath, J.H.; and Byrd, L.H., Jr. "Doctor, Brush Up Your Manners!" *RN* 46, no. 5 (May 1983): 64–65.

Sheard, T. "The Structure of Conflict in Nurse-Physician Relations." *Supervisor Nurse* 11, no. 8 (August 1980): 14–18.

Shumaker, D., and Goss, V. "Toward Collaboration: One Small Step." *Nursing Health Care* 1, no. 4 (November 1980): 183–185.

Singleton, A.F. "Physician-Nurse Perceptions of Styles of Power Usage." *Social-Sci-Med (E)* 15, no. 3 (August 1981): 231–237.

Sovik, W.E. "Physician-nurse Relationship From the Physician Viewpoint." *Ohio State Medical Journal* 76, no. 1 (January 1980): 37–38.

Stanley, I. "Accountability in Nursing. Where Do We Stand with Doctors?" *Nursing Times* 79, no. 38 (September 21–27, 1983): 46–48.

Stein, Leonard I. "The Doctor-Nurse Game." *Archives of General Psychiatry* 16 (June 1967): 699–703.

Styles, Margretta M. *On Nursing: Toward a New Endowment.* St. Louis, Mo.: C.V. Mosby Co., 1982, pp. 142–150.

Styles, Margretta M. "Reflections on Collaboration and Unification." *Image: The Journal of Nursing Scholarship* 16, no. 1 (Winter 1984): 21–23.

Sumner, E. "Time to Overturn 'Doctor's Law'." *Nursing Times* 77, no. 43 (October 28–November 3, 1981): 1874.

Torrez, Sister Mary Rachel. "Systems Approach to Staffing." *Nursing Management* 14, no. 5 (May 1983): 54.

Trinosky, P. "Nurse-doctor Dissension Still Thrives." *Supervisor Nurse* 10, no. 4 (April 1979): 40–43.

Wilson, J. "Ethics and the Physician-Nurse Relationship." *Canadian Medical Association Journal* 129, no. 3 (August 1, 1983): 290–293.

Winker, Cynthia K., and Lee, Nancy C. "Developing a Joint Practice Team." *Dimensions of Critical Care Nursing* 1, no. 6 (November/December 1982): 360–363.

Wise, Harold; Rubin, Irwin; and Beckard, Richard. "Making Health Teams Work." *American Journal of Diseases in Children* 127 (April 1974): 537–542.

Chapter 9

Nurses Interfacing with the Community

Bobbie J. Mackay, R.N., M.S.N., M.S.W.

INTRODUCTION

In the past two decades, technological advances and escalating costs of health care have altered the direction and focus of health care. These influences will shape the future direction of nursing. Nurses should view the resultant pressures as positive forces and take advantage of the opportunities for potential growth. This is a strategic time for nurses to expand the dimensions and sophistication of nursing practice. The intimate nature of their interactions with people afford nurses an opportunity to respond creatively to society's changing needs and future challenges. Opportunities for development are most prevalent in the community as there are strong pressures to shift health care delivery from tertiary care settings to the home and primary care settings. Hospitals and health care facilities will be required to develop and organize community services.

Current health care trends influence collaborative nursing interactions between health care institutions and the community. This discussion of collaborative nursing activities in the community will explore interdisciplinary approaches that facilitate the development of a more integrated, cost-effective health care system. It will describe the shift of health care delivery from institutional-based care to community and home-based care, as well as the shift in emphasis from curative, acute care to health promotion and maintenance, disease prevention, and rehabilitation. Characteristics of health care, economic and environmental trends, consumer needs, and professional and marketing issues will be discussed in relation to the effects they have on future nursing roles and the types and goals of programs and services.

CURRENT HEALTH CARE TRENDS

The current structure of health services is not responsive enough to changing illness patterns. Medicine focuses on highly specialized and sophisticated medical and surgical treatment techniques for acute conditions, while the incidence of stress-related, chronic, debilitative disease is reaching epidemic proportions. The recent development of freestanding emergency centers exemplifies this trend. In addition, the media reinforces attention to technological advances in health care by focusing on topics such as organ replacements.

Treatment and prevention of psychosocial dysfunction have progressed more slowly. Thus, clinicians are unable to assist patients and families to deal adequately with the physical, social, and psychological implications of illness. Specialization tends to fragment and depersonalize care as specialists tend to their area of expertise, ignoring other potential or existing medical concerns. Too little attention has been directed toward preventive, ambulatory, and home care services that address the needs of chronically ill individuals. Consequently, the health care system is unprepared to deal with these complex and lifelong issues.[1]

Medical costs have increased sharply as a result of inflation, increased consumer demand for and use of complex technology, inefficient management of health facilities, and patterns of insurance reimbursement. Insurance reimbursement continues to emphasize the treatment of acute care problems.[2] Private and public costs for long-term care have escalated while governmental budget restrictions have been instituted.

Health services are not distributed equally. Restrictions imposed by cost containment measures and the inequitable distribution of services seriously hinder access to services.

Consumers, no longer intimidated by health care professionals, are questioning the integrity of the system, claiming personal control, and refusing to follow medical recommendations unequivocally. As they become more knowledgeable and self-confident about their health care needs, they claim the right to participate in making decisions about their own health care. Consumers insist on greater fiscal accountability of health agencies in order to reduce the exorbitant costs of care. In addition, they are shifting their preferences for institutionally based programs to self-help and home care programs.

In addition, control over medical treatment strategies is shifting away from hospitals and physicians to the agencies and companies actually paying the bills, such as insurance companies, health maintenance organizations, Medicaid, and Medicare. In the near future, the agencies will determine access to services, types and availability of services, and reimbursement amounts. Consumers will have to decide if they are more satisfied with these agencies in control than with physicians and health personnel.

COMPONENTS OF HEALTH CARE DELIVERY

As consumer needs change and services become obsolete, the health care organization appears maladapted to its existing environment and unresponsive to its public. Changing illness patterns, consumer health care needs, the goals of services, current health care trends, and community components interrelate in a dynamic process which influences the total health care system. Alterations of one component will affect all the others.

To meet the current demands of consumers and reduce the inadequacies in health care services, nurses must become more attuned and responsive to these components. A marketing approach to health care focuses on consumer needs as a prime concern. Consumer satisfaction and welfare is the key to the success of the health care industry.[3,4]

The target population (consumers) includes individuals, families, and groups at risk for illness in the community. Health care interventions contribute to the health of consumers and reflect the needs of the total population.

The ultimate goal of health care services is to enable consumers to achieve an optimal level of physical, psychological, and social functioning. To promote satisfaction and welfare, health care professionals market integrated services and products to consumers to alleviate their difficulties and meet their health care needs. Currently, the major strategies undertaken include improving access to services and quality of care, cost-containment, alleviation of consumer stress, and reintegration of persons at risk into the community. These strategies require a design of services that address the total needs of the community as well as those of the individual. Health promotion and maintenance, disease prevention, and rehabilitation services must not only be operational but a major focus of health programs if consumer needs are to be met. Health professionals in acute care facilities must join forces with their colleagues in the community. Through interprofessional collaboration, they can provide comprehensive, coordinated, and continuous care; expand home, community-based, and self-care programs; offer diversified health programs; and influence financial reimbursement policies. Collaboration ensures that sufficient attention is given to the physical aspects of care, psychological aspects of adjustment, and social milieu of consumers.[5] Nurses can be instrumental in fostering collaboration between components of the health care system in the community.

Assessment is the foundation for program and policy planning and resource development that is responsive to consumer needs, establishes priorities for solutions, and predicts the outcomes of intervention. A comprehensive, epidemiologic analysis of the community and health care market will help identify needs and existing services. Epidemiology is concerned with the processes that influence the physical, social, and psychological health of consumers. It describes populations at risk, levels of prevention, and prevalence and incidence rates of illnesses. Target populations must be analyzed in the context of a total community study. This includes an assessment of consumer needs, the availability, accessibility, and adequacy of key resources, people, and services, the ability of existing services to expand or change, economic support systems, and environmental factors. Social implications of illness include chronicity, visibility, criticality, and predictability. Psychological implications are analyzed in terms of the nature of the illness, its effect on the level of social and independent functioning, and the extent that the total population is affected.[6] A comprehensive epidemiologic analysis of the health care market is obtained through frequent contacts between consumers and planners, personal interviews, and public surveys. It requires close collaboration between health professionals in institutional and community settings and consumers.

Once the market analysis is complete, program development and evaluation can begin. Nurses have an integrating effect in the community by enabling consumers to make better use of community resources, programs, and services and by facilitating a greater degree of response to consumers' needs on the part of the health care organization.

Nurses implement change with consumers and the environment through coordinated use of community resources. Resources and services need to be evaluated to determine how effective they are in promoting consumer satisfaction and welfare. Once nurses determine the strengths and deficits in the system, they collaborate with other community agencies and consumers to cultivate, restore, conserve, and create services and resources. They rally in response to health care demands to induce forces within the community to create new resources. For example, community action groups are emerging and gaining momentum to meet the demands of the urban scene.[7]

To meet the long-term interests of consumers, nurses should continue to collaborate with responsive resources and services during noncrisis times. This interim collaboration is expected to reduce the amount of response time on the part of health services. It also safeguards consumers' access to resources because services are offered on an ongoing basis.

COMPREHENSIVE/CONTINUOUS CARE

Comprehensive care incorporates follow-up supervision of consumers in the hospital, home, or out-patient departments during convalescence and rehabilitation.[8] It implies continuity of care, holistic care, and coordination of diverse elements of care.

Resource referral programs and discharge planning are essential components of continuity of care. The referral process identifies appropriate community resources. Discharge planning constitutes the preparations involved that ensure that consumer needs will continue to be met from one health service to another. Nurses contribute to discharge planning and resource referral by participating in multidisciplinary planning teams, developing tools to evaluate consumer discharge needs, and planning follow-up with health care resources. Discharge planning incorporates the consumer's environment, assessed needs, and available resources. Better utilization of time and personnel fosters optimum use of health services by reducing duplication of efforts. Thus careful planning reduces costs.

DIVERSIFIED HEALTH CARE PROGRAMMING

Diversified, one-stop service for consumers may be a cost-containment strategy leading to an appropriate match between consumer needs and health services. Linking acute care facilities or health maintenance organizations to community or home health agencies expands the spectrum of acute, long-term, and social services offered to consumers. Diversification increases efficiency by reducing the number of administrative personnel, the time service staff spend locating outside resources, and any organizational slack.[9] Diversification allows health agencies to provide a variety of services, such as adult day care programs, half-way houses for chronically ill adults, outpatient rehabilitation for the physically handicapped, and hospice or respite care for families with disabled or chronically ill children and elders.

HOME CARE PROGRAMS

Home care programs extend hospital services into the community for chronically ill and long-term patients and their families so that they can receive the necessary care and services at home. Home care programs, as cost containment strategies, attempt to reduce the costs of health care by limiting the length of hospitalization. Although home care places additional stress, time burdens, and responsibilities on family members, it also places control back into their hands. Home care is an important first step in rehabilitation and reintegration into the community because it fosters the development of independent functioning in consumers.

The community at this time is ill prepared to meet the mounting demands for home care. Home care programs are poorly financed and provide fragmented care that lacks the sophistication and technology of acute care facilities. Increasingly, a discrepancy is developing between the types of services consumers need and the services financed by third party payers. Thus, the competition between health agencies for limited funding is fierce. The greatest gaps in services are long-term care in the home and short-term intensive services for acute illness.[10]

In recent years there has been a marked shift in the economic backers for home health agencies from nonprofit or government agencies to for-profit organizations. These profitmaking companies provide services to persons in the community who have a source of funding available to them and avoid treating Medicaid or Medicare patients.[11]

For-profit drug and alcohol detoxification and treatment centers exemplify this concept. Increasing numbers of chemically dependent consumers and alcoholics, seeking treatment, have flooded the health care marketplace beyond its capacity to provide adequate services. A large number of these centers are profitmaking corporations. With consumer demands overburdening the health system's ability to meet these demands, centers often have long waiting lists of potential clients. As a result, these treatment centers are selective about who they treat and limit admissions primarily to consumers who have adequate sources of funding to pay for treatment. These discriminatory admission practices limit access to services and increase the inequities of care.

Although home and community-based care is considered a more cost-effective approach to health care than hospitalization, third party payers have not concurrently expanded their home care benefits. Several cost-containment strategies actually impede the use of these services. Some politicians are placing ceilings on government programs that fund home care. In addition, some of the funding sources restrict eligibility to patients that are homebound or require skilled nursing services. Patients requiring temporary services are more likely to receive assistance than those requiring long-term care. Patients awaiting placement in nursing homes are eligible for an expanded range of home health services, but others must prove that they would require hospitalization in order to obtain assistance.[12]

Home care or community-based programs cannot survive unless third party payers revise the cost containment strategies that impede the success of these programs. Nurses are in a pivotal position because of their direct experiences with the health care environments to lobby for more liberal payment strategies from third party payers for home care. However, prior to lobbying, they need to collect data that substantiate the cost effectiveness of home care. To date very little research has been completed that actually documents this claim.

IMPACT OF COST CONTAINMENT STRATEGIES

Cost containment strategies applied to the health care industry, such as prospective payment plans, health maintenance organizations, and diagnostic related groups, offer diverse opportunities for nurses to influence policy-making decisions, budget development, and resource allocation. Nurses, in response to Medicaid's tendency to limit the types and amounts of services available or to reimburse providers at low rates, should focus on searching for innovative methods of financing home or community-based health services and promoting equitable access to care.

Revising health services and programs so that they are comprehensive and well coordinated will reduce charges to funding organizations. Nurses involved in policy-making activities are better able to protect consumers from discriminatory treatment practices of for-profit organizations. These efforts work to increase access to services and reduce inequities in care.

Access to health care services can be improved by increasing programs offered by nurses and making them widely available. Direct payment for nursing services from payment resources will expand nursing roles and contain costs of care. However, agencies financing health services need greater exposure to and evidence of the cost-effective value of nurses in expanded roles, such as nurse practitioners or clinical nurse specialists. Thus, nurses in expanded roles must demonstrate their abilities and value as well as substantiate the cost effectiveness of their roles. (See Chapter 1.) Collaboration between nurses and administrators is necessary in order to analyze nursing costs and develop profiles on clinical care costs for each diagnosis and nursing unit. This information provides the justification for pricing services.

Nurses are challenged to improve the efficiency, technology, sophistication, and quality of community health care services and devise improved strategies for capturing and retaining revenue sources. Expansion of community and home-based programs offers innumerable opportunities for nurses to adopt innovative roles to provide appropriate consumer services and programs. Nurses have a great deal of flexibility in determining their roles. They may consult to troubleshoot for home health care agencies, work directly in assisting consumers solve problems, or provide education for professional associates and consumers in the community.

Nurses provide the humane operations of consumer services and contribute in a broader sense to the development and improvement of community programs and policies. Nurses enlighten various professional associates about consumer attributes and health care needs to gain their participation in program planning and implementation. Nurses collaborate with these associates to tailor programs to meet consumer needs. Collaboration provides overall consistent direction to the therapeutic programs and policies and minimizes duplication of effort or adverse competition among various agencies. It therefore is cost effective because it minimizes duplication of charges.

To provide quality care, nurses assume multiple roles: liaison, counselor, advocate, clinician, consultant, educator, team member, and program/policy planner. Each nurse uniquely implements these various professional roles and brings to each task insight into complex consumer problems and knowledge about the community and available resources.

In each of the roles identified, except that of advocate, nurses collaborate in jointly determined relationships with other professionals and consumers. They interact cooperatively in the best interest and with the permission of consumers. Their roles are defined according to the area of clinical expertise (educational and experiential qualifications), in congruence with professional practice legislation, policies of the health organization, and state laws, and in response to the needs of the community.

Nurses must be astute in choosing appropriate target populations, points of entry into consumer structures, beneficial roles, domains of functioning, and times of intervention if they are going to have a positive effect on community health care.[13] Their solutions must be acceptable to the target population. As nurses expand the scope of their practice, their success will depend upon whether they have properly prepared for roles that are both beneficial and marketable in the future health care scene.

LIAISONS

Nurses, as intermediaries, collaborate with consumers, other health care personnel, or agencies in order to implement changes that would improve the consumer's life situation. The role of liaison presumes a complementary link and mutuality of purpose among consumers, health personnel, and the community. An exchange of services and goods takes place in the health care marketplace that is mutually beneficial to both groups of participants: the seeker receives the requested support and reinforcement through the services received; the provider (seller) usually receives financial payment for services and personal gratification that comes with meeting the needs of others.[14,15]

Consumers vary in their ability to deal independently with community resources and services. Consequently, nurses apply different levels of intervention to the referral process. The ultimate goal is to assist consumers to utilize resources independently and accept responsibility for meeting their own health care needs. Some consumers need assistance dealing with all aspects of problem-solving processes and/or referral or resource utilization processes while others require little assistance.

Nursing interventions with consumers unable to function independently involves health teaching related to disease prevention, availability of affordable resources, or appropriate utilization of resources and services. It involves counseling, planning for home care needs, and providing support so that health needs can be identified and appropriate referrals made. Initially, nurses may need to assist some consumers in making most of their arrangements for health care. It is tempting and frequently easier for nurses to do the work for consumers rather than to facilitate self-care.

Professionals who do the work for consumers interfere with the consumers' independent functioning. This reinforces future dependency in the utilization of services and resources and inadvertently places the responsibility for health care on professionals. Consumer dependency on health care personnel interferes with the provision of cost-effective care and places unnecessary physical and financial burdens on the health care system.

A large number of chronically ill adults pose serious adjustment problems that have exceeded the community's capacity to deal with them. Those individuals are misfits in the community with nowhere to go and few family or community resources to provide appropriate and adequate assistance. They seek some semblance of independent living and yet require assistance with activities of daily living, that is, food preparation, paying bills and budgeting, or following through with the treatment regimen prescribed for their medical condition.

Recently, I assisted a 32-year-old man with cystic fibrosis, John, who exemplifies this problem. John had multiple physical and emotional problems to contend with: progressive obstructive lung disease, diabetes secondary to cystic fibrosis, malnutrition, and depression. In addition, he manifested a thought disorder bordering on paranoid schizophrenia. John's only living relatives were unwilling to assist him in any way. Even though his psychiatric disorder was borderline, through close collaboration with professional associates from a hospital-based pulmonary program and a psychiatric community placement program, he was able to find enough financial assistance from state and federal programs to provide funds for food, shelter, and miscellaneous needs. He was also able to find a suitable place to live with close access to inexpensive restaurants and the medical facility where he received his care. Until he had a good understanding of how to care for himself and was compliant with the medical regimen, a visiting nurse regularly called on him to assess his needs, draw up his insulin, and evaluate his eating habits. Eventually, through vocational rehabilitation, John was able to find part-time employment, which enabled him to be more financially self-reliant.

This example demonstrates three key points necessary for the provision of consumer-oriented health care. First, existing resources and services in the community need to be flexible in their eligibility requirements to include persons who fail to fit rigid standards. Existing programs need to modify their format or goals to meet the new needs of the marketplace. Second, hospital personnel need to extend into the community and collaborate regularly with professional associates to concentrate their efforts into a strong workforce, reduce duplication of effort, improve marketing strategies, and provide comprehensive, cost-effective programs. Third, additional resources, programs, and services need to be developed to meet the new demands for health care.

Currently, resources are inadequate, underutilized, and financially unstable. In order to develop new facets or improve existing circumstances, these resources need to be converted into useful programs and distributed efficiently to consumers. Proposals for future community placement programs should include accommodations, medical supervision, and funding for the large numbers of the chronically ill, the mentally retarded adults, and the elderly.

COUNSELING

Counseling enables consumers to confront stressful situations and search for information and causative factors. Counselors assist consumers to explore alternative ways of handling stress or solving problems. Counselors apply principles of stress management to help consumers reduce levels of stress, resolve crises, and prepare for dealing with future difficulties. Principles of conflict resolution and teaching-learning are applied to develop consumers' cognitive, motor, and affective skills. Consumers learn skills that enhance their problem-solving capabilities, help them make informed decisions, and motivate alteration of their behavior. They subsequently take progressive responsibility for their own behavior or decisions.[16]

Consumers apply problem-solving techniques to identify and clarify the nature of their problems, break crisis events into smaller, more manageable issues, explore alternative solutions, and make decisions based on their best options.[17] They experience improved interpersonal skills and a greater sense of independence, self-confidence, and self-determination as they manage difficulties.

Nurses engage in four levels of counseling: preventive, evaluative, problem-oriented, and supportive. Preventive counseling provides anticipatory guidance to prevent excessive guilt or maladaptive behavior. Evaluative counseling identifies current consumer problems and determines the extent of unmet needs. Supportive counseling encourages ventilation of feelings and experiences. Counselors strive to enhance consumer self-esteem and self-confidence by demonstrating confidence in their ability to overcome difficulties and giving positive reinforcement. Problem-oriented counseling facilitates problem-solving activities and enhances consumer problem-solving abilities.

The temptation for counselors to assume "rescue" behavior by giving advice and/or making decisions for consumers is very seductive, especially for counselors in rehabilitation or chronic illness programs who interact closely with consumers for sustained periods of time. Rescue tactics have the same consequences for consumers, whether professionals merely give advice or actually perform a task that consumers are responsible for. Rescuing temporarily reduces consumer anxiety but, in the long run, encourages dependency on professionals and leaves consumers unprepared to deal with difficulties in the future.

GROUP WORK

Group work is especially valuable in helping patients and families cope with the emotional and social implications of illness. Groups provide mutual support, acceptance, universalization, reality testing, socialization, task accomplishment, and hope. These provisions meet the needs of people experiencing a disruption in their interpersonal relationships. Groups assist members to face and deal with the social realities of living with an illness and with their emotional reactions.[18] The idea of mutual support and assistance implies a process of give and take; each member learns from and gives to others. If the group is effective, members progress from various levels of dependency to develop greater independence and self-reliance.

Groups are categorized by their purposes, goals, and utilization. Examples of groups include: educational, therapeutic, self-help, social-change, team, and training groups. Educational groups share knowledge and competence in areas of common interest among members. Therapeutic groups assist members to gain personal insight and change behaviors interfering with their personal development. These groups relieve the social isolation members experience and enhance their ability to cope with illness and subsequent role changes.[19] Self-help groups aim to control socially unacceptable behavior of members such as substance abuse, child abuse, or overeating; provide peer support and mutual aid to cope with stress; and improve member self-esteem by overcoming public discrimination.

Social-change groups are task oriented and seek modification of some aspect of the health care system. The goals of social-change groups are achieved through collective problem solving by consumers. This form of self-help group deals with issues on a global level. Human relations training groups promote the psychosocial development of participants. Individuals attend training groups for the purpose of learning cognitive and affective characteristics of human relations.[20]

Group activity is being recognized as an important therapeutic approach to health care. Nurses need to incorporate group work as a method of intervention. The outcomes of group process are dependent on the competence and knowledge of the group leader. Nurses with knowledge and skill in group process should apply their expertise in conducting training, educational, and/or therapeutic groups to promote the psychosocial and physical health of community members. Group work in the past was dominated by social workers and was primarily therapeutic in nature. Nurses now have more opportunities to be involved in group work as they interface with the community health care system. They should organize ideas and plans for groups and market them in the health care system. As more demands are placed on the health care system, group activity provides a means of reaching a larger number of people than individual intervention and is therefore cost effective. These groups produce revenue for the sponsoring agencies and opportunities for nurses to expand their roles and scope of practice.

Therapeutic groups of individuals with chronic illness or parents of individuals with chronic illness are usually more successful if discussions incorporate a blend of didactic information about the illness with psychosocial issues. Nurses, with knowledge of illness, medical treatment, and psychosocial issues, are natural candidates for conducting groups of this nature. Examples of popular groups that serve consumers include parent effectiveness training, stress management, assertiveness training, sexuality workshops, and relaxation groups.

HEALTH EDUCATION

Health education is an integral part of health care. Hospitals and other health care institutions form the network responsible for providing comprehensive health education programs. Accomplishment of this task requires close coordination and collaboration among hospitals, health care institutions, community agencies, and motivated consumers. Collaboration enables health care professionals to clarify their roles and responsibilities for health education; identify consumer needs; exchange professional knowledge, insights, and values; and plan and implement health education programs. It minimizes the risks of duplicating professional efforts or deleting important programs.

Currently, health education focuses on illness and is practiced primarily in hospital settings; thus patients get the most concentrated educational services. Health education emphasizes health promotion, which includes health maintenance, rehabilitation, disease and trauma management, preventive health practices, and proper health care utilization practices. It incorporates two major components: (1) acquisition of knowledge to increase consumer's understanding of situations and (2) application of acquired information. Health education relates information about specific disease conditions, treatment approaches, prognosis, financial resources, physical limitations, medications, and home care treatment plans.[21]

Health education prepares consumers to deal more constructively with developmental and situational events, practice personal habits that foster optimal health, and manage stress so that they can concentrate their energy on achievement of their goals. This includes preparation for procedures, tests, or surgery. A common program offered in pediatric health settings is the pre-admission party. This program exemplifies prevention through preparation as it prepares children for hospitalization prior to admission.

The recipients of health education are patients and families, health personnel, and the community at large. Nurses should recognize the opportunity to implement a leadership role in health education that reaches all three targets. They can be central to the development of marketable health education programs in the community. Health education stresses individual responsibility for protecting health and the importance of health care in reducing the incidence of illness, disease, and injury. With the self-care market growing, educational programs that teach people how to exercise responsibility for self-care must be developed.

Educational programs that emphasize health promotion, disease prevention, and self care include dental hygiene, well-baby care, diet and nutrition, responsible babysitting, exercising to health, hazards of smoking, accidents and provision of a safe home environment, first aid, preparing a child for hospitalization, and immunizations. Other examples include self-care diagnostic screening programs, such as hypertension programs or breast self-examination programs. Nurses can develop and market programs that develop the personal strengths of participants for other health personnel or businesses in the community. These programs may include behavior modification training, assertiveness training, relaxation technique, and motivational dynamics.

Outreach health education programs for consumers, health care personnel, or professional associates in the community (i.e., school teachers, clergy) improve access to health facilities as well as utilization of services. By stressing the interrelatedness of physical and psychosocial aspects of illness, these health education programs remove barriers to resource utilization and continuity of care, expand opportunities for prevention and rehabilitation, and increase the public's awareness of illness-related psychosocial stresses.[22] A consciousness-raising health education program offered to school teachers across the state or nation could address the implications of chronic illness or invisible handicaps on patients and families and reduce the illness-related problems children experience at school.

ADVOCACY

An advocate identifies with the plight of the disadvantaged, pleads their causes, and protects their rights. The role of advocate assumes that a situational conflict exists between consumers and social or environmental resources. Consumers are represented as victims being unjustly treated or deprived of access and resources.[23]

Nurses, through their frequent contacts with the environment and consumers, become acutely aware of the deficiencies in the health care system. They are frequently tempted to adopt the advocacy role. Yet, advocacy will potentially escalate rather than alleviate consumer difficulties.

Four major dilemmas are associated with the advocate role: (1) conflicting loyalty, (2) adversary response, (3) temporary appeasement, and (4) domination of consumers. Conflicting loyalties develop when values that stress a primary obligation to consumers conflict with the institutional obligations of the professional. Ideally, consumers take priority over employers.[24] Realistically, however, professionals advocating against their own organization risk jeopardizing organizational activities and losing their jobs.

The adversary response refers to a defensive reaction often conveyed in response to an advocate. Individuals assume roles that either complement or interfere with the roles of others. If advocacy is viewed as interference or criticism, it can provoke an adversary response. This response inhibits communication and interferes with positive action in the consumer's interest.

Temporary appeasement refers to the palliative effects of advocacy. It represents the classic dilemma of which needs should be met, those of the individual or those of society.[25] Resolution of one individual's difficulties may jeopardize the effectiveness of resources offered to a larger group of consumers.

The fourth dilemma, domination of consumers, occurs when health care providers accept too much responsibility for consumers and take over consumer action. This tendency to dominate has the same repercussions for consumers as rescuing or giving advice.[26]

Nurses should implement advocacy only when total conflict of interest develops between resource and consumer. Nurses accomplish more on behalf of consumers and minimize detrimental outcomes if they interact cooperatively with other providers than if they advocate against the other providers. Endorsement of advocacy should be tempered to restrain the tendency to dominate. Efforts should be rechanneled to link consumers with available resources and services. If a breakdown occurs, nurses can mediate to change ways in which consumers and service personnel deal with each other.[27] When other strategies have been unsuccessful, however, nurses may have no alternative but to assume the advocate role. Advocacy may be implemented either by acting for consumers or by teaching them to advocate for themselves. With either application of this role, nurses have a responsibility to inform consumers, prior to intervention, of the potential negative consequences. Consumers should then make their own decision about whether to risk the untoward consequences of the advocate approach.

Once professionals have applied the advocate role, they should try to alter conditions to minimize the necessity of repeating that role. They should extensively study the deficits in the system responsible for the conflict. Then, they should collaborate with the previous adversary to modify the system so that, in the future, consumer rights would be upheld without intervention from an advocate.[28] The result is a positive contribution rather than repeated conflicts.

THE CONSULTANT ROLE

The role of consultant has many applications for nurses in the community health care system. Consultation is an interactional process of shared thinking that involves the assistance of a specialist in relation to a problem. The consultant offers specialized knowledge and insight to improve the management of a problem and to enhance the skill of consultees in managing similar situations in the future.[29]

Consultation is applied to effect change in individuals, families, groups, or programs. The process and techniques of consultation are similar in each situation, but the content will vary widely depending on the consultees' needs and the consultant's expertise. Consultees identify the problem and recognize it as being within the consultant's area of expertise. The consultant offers clarification, interpretation, and education in relation to the identified problem. Consultees then have the responsibility for making final decisions about what action is taken and for implementing this action. They are free to accept or reject the consultant's suggestions.[30]

The consultant assists in the identification of variables contributing to the problem and creates a climate for problem solving. Too much emphasis on didactic information can obscure the purpose of the consultation. The solution is likely to be more practical and easier to comply with if the consultee has been involved with the problem-solving process. In addition, identification of educational needs in the course of consultation serves as a basis for the development of future programs.

There are four types of consultation. In practice any one of them is rarely applied as a pure form but rather as part of a synthesis. The types of consultation are (1) consultee-centered case consultation, (2) client-centered case consultation, (3) program-centered administrative consultation, and (4) consultee-centered administrative consultation.[31] Case consultation involves offering assistance in the management of patients, families, or groups. In consultee-centered case consultation, the consultant works with the consultee to overcome personal deficits. In client-centered case consultation, the consultant assists the consultee by identifying available psychosocial resources and by problem solving to improve services.[32]

Program consultation addresses agency or community needs and provides assistance with issues such as staff motivation/development, new program development, availability of funding resources, and administrative efficiency. In program-centered administrative consultation, the work problem is related either to developing a new program, improving an existing program, or evaluating the effectiveness of any changes. In consultee-centered administrative consultation the problems of the consultee that interfere with the organization are identified.[33]

Three major elements significant in conducting program consultations are (1) analysis of the organization of programs in the problem-formulation stage, (2) incorporation of the health program objectives as part of the consultation objectives, and (3) assessment of forces that enhance or impede achievement of the objectives.[34]

Consultation is an effective method of expanding the role of nurses by creating opportunities for mutual and innovative problem solving, identifying values, and sharing information. Currently, the consultant role is loosely defined and underutilized. Informal contacts with physicians and other health professionals occur daily and provide an excellent starting point for more formal and organized consultation. Opportunities exist for nurses to offer consultation as an important marketable health care service in the community. It is a strategy that can bring about change in individuals and institutions to improve health care programs. Nurses expand their opportunities for providing ongoing or time-limited consultations by maintaining contact with other health care professionals within their institution or the community.

MULTIDISCIPLINARY TEAMS

Nurses participate in multidisciplinary teams to comprehend and serve consumer needs, search for solutions to consumer and community problems, and enhance the team's capacity to effect progressive change in community services and policies. A health care team is composed of a group of professionals from various educational and experiential backgrounds and consumers who share a common purpose and mutual goals. Team members collaborate regularly to share data, knowledge, and opinions; consolidate expertise; and reach joint decisions. Their collaborative efforts identify problems, determine actions, initiate programs, and outline future goals.[35] Each team member offers particular expertise and has equal obligation and involvement in the decision-making process. Team activity reflects a complementarity of efforts among members that determines its effectiveness. Each member learns to appreciate and respect the contributions of other members.

Cohesiveness is an essential component of productive teamwork. It develops over time as team members work together in a climate of acceptance, flexibility, and understanding. Each member must be aware of and tend to the emotional, intellectual, and professional needs of other members to promote constructive interaction. Teams balance the influences of member values and goals, consumer needs and rights, and overall community health objectives in the process of planning.

Insights gained through collaboration with team members enable nurses to look beyond the urgent needs of the individual to the common aspects of need in the community. Nurses clarify and interpret the information obtained about community dynamics and needs to other professionals on the team. In addition, they interpret the type of assistance the team has to offer and clarify the functions of each member.

Consumer participation on health care teams as equal partners with health professionals reduces the powerlessness consumers experience in dealing with health care systems, improves their level of compliance, and safeguards consumer need satisfaction. Consumer participation permits accurate assessment of consumer needs, identification of needed programs and services, and establishment of a consumer communication network.

COMMUNITY PLANNING

Nurses must extend their collaborative efforts with consumers and health care teams to include community organizations so that they have opportunities to contribute to community program and policy development. They participate on multidisciplinary teams to formulate, implement, and evaluate community programs and policies.

Community planning occurs at local, state, and national levels through different modalities such as social, voluntary, and governmental. It occurs in different fields of practice such as rehabilitation, welfare, or health. Nurses are responsible for understanding the immediate and long-term effects of programs they develop on consumers and the community. They are being asked to participate in the planning of a growing number of new health programs related to chronic illness, alcoholism, industrial health, and drug rehabilitation programs.

EXPANDING ROLES OF NURSES

The roles of master's prepared clinicians and nurse practitioners evolved in the 1960s and 1970s in response to current health care trends. These roles developed to improve the quality of nursing care, and they continue to evolve in response to changing health care needs.

Nurse practitioners extended into the community health field to deliver primary health care directly to well populations. Initially they filled a need by replacing a shortage of physicians in the community. This shortage opened up many opportunities for nurses to try new approaches. Their plans were implemented through independent action, appropriate referrals, health counseling and teaching, and collaboration with other health care providers. Problems of primary prevention, monitoring chronic conditions, and alleviation of situational or developmental stress are within the realm of the nurse practitioner's expertise.[36]

Master's prepared clinicians have practiced primarily in tertiary care settings. Currently the role is expanding in the community either as an extension of tertiary care centers or in a new capacity as community health clinical specialists. The relative flexibility, autonomy, and availability that clinical specialists experience in their practices contribute to the effectiveness of this clinical role. These same characteristics may interfere with the acceptance and recognition of clinical specialists by other health personnel because they perpetuate the ambiguity associated with the role. Consistent, productive contact with staff and consumers lends credence to the validity and significance of this clinical role. Master's prepared clinicians provide support, education, referrals, and long-term followup services to patients and families. In addition, much of their time is devoted to educating, consulting with, and counseling professional colleagues, or to implementing research.

Clinical specialists and nurse practitioners address consumer needs and intervene strategically to alleviate gaps of care. They facilitate optimal use of services and resources, improve coordination of services and programs, and participate in program and policy planning for health care in the community. In the last decade, nurse practitioners have become established in the community health care system. The boundaries for master's prepared clinicians are less clearly defined. Perceptions that other health professionals develop about nurse clinicians will influence their acceptance by the community in the future. These clinicians need to develop marketing strategies in the community to alter any ambiguous images and to build positive attitudes that reflect quality patient and family care.

SUMMARY

Currently, economic conditions and health care trends have placed increasing demands on health care providers. Traditionally, nurses have been portrayed in a "helping" role in which they take care of people. However, the demands on the health care system to provide acute and primary care and to expand preventive, rehabilitation, and long-term care services are so great that nurses can no longer afford to focus narrowly on meeting the individual needs of consumers. Instead, they must take a more global approach and consider the total health care picture of consumers in the community. Nurses in tertiary and community care settings must combine forces with each other and diversify their programs in order to meet the changing needs of consumers more effectively. Collaboration between these health care elements protects the survival of the various institutions, agencies, or services in the health care market place. In this manner, nurses can offer more organized and efficient services to absorb health care responsibilities and can offer these services to larger groups of consumers.

Self-sufficiency of consumers in dealing with the health care system should be fostered to reduce some of the demands on personnel. Nurses intervene to improve the consumer's cognitive and motor skills, problem-solving capabilities, and understanding of community resources and services. Consumers are then able to utilize these components more appropriately and effectively.

The roles nurses implement in the context of community interaction affect their public images and their acceptance as health care providers. They should facilitate collaboration with other health care professionals by assuming complementary roles. At times, however, nurses involved in program or policy planning may need to challenge community establishments or authorities for the good of the community at large. Their strategies may have political connotations, controversial components, or unorthodox characteristics. Assuming responsibility for planning programs and policies is not an approach of least resistance, but it is a professional responsibility that should be accepted seriously. Nurses should avail themselves of the opportunities to participate in program and policy planning so that they can influence the direction of health care and nursing in the future, instead of accepting the consequences from the planning of others.

The issues of accountability and liability will be of primary importance as nurses assume expanded roles in health care institutions or in the community. Presently, no precedent has been set and little information is available that addresses these issues. Since there are potential risks in assuming expanded roles and greater responsibility in health care, the issues of accountability and liability are areas that need further thought and consideration.

NOTES

1. Neil F. Bract, *Social Work in Health Care: A Guide to Professional Practice* (New York: Haworth Press, 1978), pp. 37–49.

2. Ibid.

3. P. Kotler, *Marketing for Non-Profit Organizations* (Englewood Cliffs, N.J.: Prentice Hall, Inc., 1975), p. 47.

4. R.E. MacStravic, *Marketing Health Care* (Rockville, Md.: Aspen Systems Corp., 1977).

5. Harriet M. Bartlett, *Social Work Practice in the Health Field* (Washington, D.C.: National Association of Social Workers, 1961), pp. 60–66.

6. Bertha L. Doremus, "The Four Rs: Social Diagnosis in Health Care," *Health and Social Work* 1, no. 4 (1976): 121–139.

7. Ruth Middleman and Gale Goldberg, *Social Service Delivery: A Structural Approach to Social Work Practice* (New York: Columbia University Press, 1974), pp. 54–65.

8. P. Snoke and E.R. Weinerman, "Comprehensive Care Programs in University Medical Centers," *Journal of Medical Education*, July 1965, pp. 625–657.

9. Gary R. Summers, "Economics of Successful Health Maintenance Organizations," *Nursing Economics* 1 (November–December 1983): 385–390.

10. J.B. Wood and C.L. Estes, "Home Health Care Under the Policies of New Federalism," *Caring* 3, no. 6 (1984): 58–61.

11. Ibid.

12. Laura Reif, "Making Dollars and Sense of Home Health Policy," *Nursing Economics* 2 (November/December 1984): 382–385.

13. Max Siporin, "Social Treatment: A New-Old Helping Method," *Social Work* (July 1970): 22–23.

14. Ruth Middleman and Gale Goldberg, *Social Service Delivery: A Structural Approach to Social Work Practice* (New York: Columbia University Press, 1974), pp. 54–59.

15. Ann B. Hamric, "Role Development and Functions," *The Clinical Nurse Specialist in Theory and Practice,* ed. Ann B. Hamric and Judy Spross (New York: Grune and Stratton, 1983), pp. 40–44.

16. S.A. Clemen, D.G. Eigsti, and S.L. McGuire, *Comprehensive Family and Community Health Nursing* (New York: McGraw-Hill Book Company, 1981), pp. 186–187.

17. Ruth Beckman Murray and Judith Proctor Zentner, *Nursing Concepts for Health Promotion,* 2nd ed. (Englewood Cliffs; N.J.: Prentice-Hall, Inc., 1979), pp. 291–337.

18. Ibid., pp. 189–194.

19. M.E. Loomis, *Group Process for Nurses.* (St. Louis, Mo.: C.V. Mosby Co., 1979), pp. 3–11.

20. Harriet M. Bartlett, *Social Work Practice in the Health Field* (Washington, D.C.: National Association of Social Workers, 1961), pp. 206–210.

21. Barbara Klug Redman, *The Process of Patient Teaching in Learning.* 3rd ed. (St. Louis, Mo.: The C.V. Mosby Co., 1976), p. 27.

22. Neil F. Bract, *Social Work in Health Care: A Guide to Professional Practice* (New York: Haworth Press, 1978), pp. 21–24.

23. Ruth Middleman and Gale Goldberg, *Social Service Delivery: A Structural Approach to Social Work Practice* (New York: Columbia University Press, 1974), pp. 54–59.

24. Linda M. Claxton, "Advocacy: An Application in Children," *Social Work in Education* (Washington, D.C.: National Association of Social Workers, 1981), p. 46.

25. Ibid., pp. 47–48.

26. Ibid., p. 47.

27. Ibid., pp. 43–54.

28. Ruth Middleman and Gale Goldberg, *Social Service Delivery: A Structural Approach to Social Work Practice* (New York: Columbia University Press, 1974), p. 57.

29. Lydia Rapoport, ed., *Consultation in Social Work Practice* (New York: National Association of Social Workers, 1963), p. 18.

30. Anne-Marie Barron, "The CNS as Consultant," in *The Clinical Nurse Specialist in Theory and Practice,* ed. Ann B. Hamric and Judy Spross (New York: Grune and Stratton, 1983), pp. 91–113.

31. Ibid.

32. Neil F. Bract, *Social Work in Health Care: A Guide to Professional Practice* (New York: Haworth Press, 1978), pp. 233–235.

33. Ibid.

34. Ibid.

35. Jane Isaacs Lowe and Marjatta Herranen, "Conflict in Team Work: Understanding Roles and Relationships," *Social Work in Health Care* 3, no. 3 (Spring 1978): 324–326.

36. L. Ford and H. Silver, "Expanded Role of Nurse in Child Care," *Nursing Outlook* 15 (1967): 43–45.

SUGGESTED READINGS

Bartlett, Harriet M. *Social Work Practice in the Health Field.* Washington, D.C.: National Association of Social Workers, 1961.

Bion, W.R. *Experiences in Groups.* New York: Basic Books, 1959.

Blake, Patricia. "The Clinical Specialist as Nurse Consultant." *Journal of Nursing Administration,* December 1977, pp. 33–37.

Bloom, B.L., and Parod, H.J. "Interdisciplinary Training and Interdisciplinary Functioning: A Survey of Attitudes and Practices in Community Mental Health." *American Journal of Orthopsychiatry* 46 no. 4 (October 1976): 669–677.

Bract, Neil, F. *Social Work in Health Care: A Guide to Professional Practice.* New York: Haworth Press, 1978.

Brill, N.I. *Working With People: The Helping Process.* Philadelphia: J.B. Lippincott, 1978.

Brown, Sarah Jo. "Administrative Support" in *The Clinical Nurse Specialist in Theory and Practice.* Ed. Ann B. Hamric and Judy Spross. New York: Grune and Stratton, 1983.

Cadden, V. "Crisis in the Family." In *Principles of Preventive Psychiatry.* Ed. G. Caplan, New York: Basic Books, 1964.

Castronouo, F. "The Effective Use of the Clinical Specialist." *Supervisor Nurse* 6, no. 5 (1975): 48–56.

Claxton, Linda M. "Advocacy: An Application to Children." *Social Work in Education.* Washington, D.C.: National Association of Social Workers, 1981, pp. 43–54.

Clemen, Susan Ann; Eigsti, Diane Gerber; and McGuire, Sandra L. *Comprehensive Family and Community Health Nursing.* New York: McGraw-Hill Book Company, 1981.

Coleman, Jules V. "Collaboration, Consultation, and Referral in an Integrated Mental Health Program at an H.M.O." *Social Work in Health Care* 5 (Fall 1979): 83–96.

Doremus, Bertha L. "The Four R's: Social Diagnosis in Health Care." *Health and Social Work* 1, no. 4 (November 1976): 121–137.

Freyman, John G. *The American Health Care System: Its Genesis and Trajectory.* New York: Medcom, 1974.

Gordon, M. "The Clinical Specialist as Change Agent." *Nursing Outlook* 17, no. 3 (1969): 37–39.

Hamric, Ann B., and Spross, Judy, eds. *The Clinical Nurse Specialist in Theory and Practice.* New York: Grune and Stratton, 1983.

Hardy, M., and Conway, M., eds. *Role Theory Perspectives for Health Professionals.* New York: Appleton-Century-Crofts, 1978.

Hasenfeld, Yeheskel, and English, Richard A., eds. *Human Service Organizations.* Ann Arbor, Mich.: The University of Michigan Press, 1977.

Howard, J. "Liaison Nursing." *Journal of Psychiatric Nursing and Mental Health Services* 16, no. 4 (1978): 35–37.

Lister, Larry. "Role Expectations of Social Workers and Other Health Professionals." *Health and Social Work* 5 (May 1980): 41–49.

Loomis, M.E. *Group Process for Nurses.* St. Louis, Mo.: C.V. Mosby Co., 1979.

Loubeau, Patricia R. "Marketing as a Health Concept." *Nursing Economics* 2 (January-February 1984): 37–41.

Lowe, Jane Isaacs, and Herranen, Marjatta. "Conflict in Teamwork: Understanding Roles and Relationships." *Social Work in Health Care* 3, no. 3 (Spring 1978): 323–330.

Middleman, Ruth, and Goldberg, Gale. *Social Service Delivery: A Structural Approach to Social Work Practice.* New York: Columbia University Press, 1974.

Minahan, Anne, and Pincus, Allen. "Conceptual Framework for Social Work Practice." *Social Work* 22 (September 1977).

Murray, Ruth Beckman, and Zentner, Judith Proctor. *Nursing Concepts for Health Promotion,* 2nd ed. Englewood Cliffs, N.J.: Prentice-Hall, Inc., 1979.

Pierce, S.F., and Thompson, D. "Changing Practice: By Choice Rather than Chance." *Journal of Nursing Administration* 6, no. 2 (1976): 33–39.

Pinkerton, P. "Psychological Problems of Children with Chronic Illness." *The Care of Children With Chronic Illness, Proceedings of the 67th Conference on Pediatric Research.* Columbus, Ohio: Ross Laboratories, 1974.

Rapoport, Lydia. "The Concept of Prevention in Social Work." *Social Work* 6 (January 1961): 3–12.

Redman, Barbara K. *The Process of Patient Teaching.* St. Louis, Mo.: C.V. Mosby Co., 1976.

Reif, Linda. "Making Dollars and Sense of Home Health Policy." *Nursing Economics* 2 (November–December 1984): 382–385.

Satir, Virginia; Stackowish, James; and Taschman, Harvey. *Helping Families to Change.* New York: Jason Aronson, Co., 1975.

Schein, E.H. *Process Consultation: Its Role in Organization Development.* Reading, Mass.: Addison-Wesley Publishing Company, 1969.

Snoke, P., and Weinerman, E.R. "Comprehensive Care Programs in University Medical Centers." *Journal of Medical Education,* July 1976, pp. 625–657.

Summers, Gary R. "Economics of Successful Health Maintenance Organizations." *Nursing Economics* 1 (November–December 1983): 385–390.

Wood, J.B., and Estes, C.L. "Home Health Care Under the Policies of New Federalism." *Caring* 3, no. 6 (1984): 58–61.

Part IV

Chapter 10

Future Directions of Collaborative Practice

Carol Hill Luckey, R.N., M.S.N. (Research)

INTRODUCTION

The previous chapters have discussed various aspects of collaborative practice for professional nurses. This chapter will describe changes within the health care system and society, how the nursing profession is and will be affected by these changes, and how nurses may be utilizing collaboration in the future.

CHANGE

The future cannot be discussed without considering change. Change is inevitable and a natural part of life. According to Webster, change is to make a difference in the state or condition of a thing or to substitute another state or condition.[1] Mauksch and Miller state, "Change is the process by which alterations occur in the function and structure of society."[2]

The theory of change was first developed by the social psychologist, Kurt Lewin.[3] This theory describes individuals as dynamic, growing, social beings. Individuals and groups are affected by change even though neither may be the target of the change process. In an analysis of change theory, two frameworks will be presented: force field analysis and stages of change.

Force field analysis is a technique for determining two opposing forces: driving forces and restraining forces.[4] Driving forces are those pushing for the desired direction of change, while the restraining forces are holding back the subject of change. When no change is in progress, the opposing forces are in balance.

It is the driving forces one usually considers when effecting planned change; that is, one considers what one needs to do to accomplish the planned change. In using force field analysis, consideration of the restraining forces can reduce the restraining forces, and change is more likely to succeed.

Change theory can also be analyzed by progressing through the three stages of change process: (1) unfreezing, (2) moving, and (3) refreezing.[5] Unfreezing is the breaking down of the old ways, the old customs, the old traditions of an individual, group, or organization. The second stage, moving, is assisting in the actual change of behavior by providing education, advice, or equipment necessary to do things a new way. The moving stage cannot occur until the unfreezing stage is accomplished. The third stage, refreezing, is the process by which newly acquired behavior comes to be integrated as a regular behavior for the individual, group, or organization.

Communication is the key to both of these change theories. Information provides the rationale for change, but it is not the source of motivation for change. The motivation for change comes from the concept of problem solving. The problem-solving technique has a series of steps. First, the problem is identified. Awareness of an existing problem and the possibility of change must be known. Second, enough data is collected to analyze the problem. This will determine the exact nature of the problem. The next step is to determine all possible solutions to the problem. It is helpful here to assess the environment and the resistance to change.

The fourth step is selecting the plan for the intervention of the problem based on the possible solutions. Preparation of alternative solutions is necessary, as well as a start-up date. Implementation of the planned change, the fifth step, is then begun. The change process can be enhanced by involving participation of those affected by the change.

The sixth step is the evaluation of the change process itself. Has the change solved the problem? The answer to this question will determine if the series of steps needs to be repeated.

Many nurses are familiar with this problem-solving technique. Individualized, goal-directed nursing care is provided to patients using the four components of the nursing process: (1) assessment, (2) planning, (3) intervention, and (4) evaluation. To accomplish the nursing process, nurses utilize the problem-solving technique.

Change Within the Nursing Profession

The nursing profession has always been involved in change. Most changes for nursing, though, have been unplanned, or as a reaction to the environment, medical care, the economy, technology, or consumers. An historical perspective of nursing explains this.

Florence Nightingale became involved in nursing as a result of deplorable sanitary conditions and a war in which injured soldiers were left to die due to lack of medical care. Florence Nightingale reacted to the environment and the consumers. Through her leadership, services were provided by a corps of trained nurses. Resistance to change was a frequent occurrence, as the military personnel resented Nightingale's authority and the fact that she was a civilian and a woman.

Early nursing was practiced in patients' homes in the form of private duty nursing. Nurses were employed by a patient or the family at the discretion of the patient's physician. The physician directed and ordered all the care the nurse provided to the patient. The nurse was also the housekeeper, dietitian, florist, laundress, and anything else requested by the patient and family. Nurses reacted to physicians and consumers.

Following World War II, the environment for nursing practice changed from the consumer's home to the hospital. Technological advances and the lack of trained nurses created this change. Physicians continued to direct and order all the care the nurse provided to the patient. The nurse was required to function as the housekeeper, dietitian, florist, laundress, pharmacist, and anything else as requested by the hospital administration. Nurses reacted to physicians and administrators.

As a result of the 1948 Brown report, liberal education for nurses began to be stressed.[6] Academic tracks were available in nursing administration, supervision, and teaching. Promotions for nurses were limited to administrative or academic routes. In the 1960s, the clinical nurse specialist role developed as a reaction to a system that had forced nurses away from patients. The clinical nurse specialist's role provided nursing with the responsibility, for the first time, for health maintenance of well clients. Nursing had found its way back to the bedside and into the home and community.

Change Within the Health Care System

In the past, technology and the scientific era in medicine brought about an increase in the number of hospitals and changes in the hospitals' patterns of use. From the charity hospitals of the mid-nineteenth century evolved capital-intensive centers of medical specialization. At the turn of the twentieth century hospitals faced a financial crisis: a decrease in philanthropic and public charity incomes and at the same time an increase in expenses due to the need for equipment demanded by medical science and the influx of sicker patients. The patient population was shifting from poor to middle class, with the main source of hospital income shifting from contributions to patient fees.[7]

For the past 30 years the health care system has been largely funded by third party payers and, since 1965, Medicare and Medicaid. Public Law

98-21, enacted in 1983, created dramatic changes in the health care system. The retrospective payment policy based on costs was changed to a prospective payment policy based on the patients' diagnoses or diagnosis-related groups. The change in the payment policy was precipitated by congressional concern over the federal deficit and the fear of the Medicare trust fund going broke. The federal government will no longer pay for rising health care costs. Several reasons for rising health care costs include population changes, the effects of supply and demand, new technology, and intensity of service.[8] As a result of prospective payment systems (shorter length of stays) hospitals are experiencing a decline in patient census. This has resulted in hospitals becoming competitive. Marketing directors have become key employees in hospitals, with advertising of services one of the new marketing strategies.

Nationally, the economics of the health care system will continue to change. The American College of Hospital Administrators together with Arthur Anderson and Company conducted a study to determine the consensus of health care experts concerning the future direction of the health care system.[9] Data were categorized into seven broad areas: (1) social philosophy, (2) regulations, (3) payment systems, (4) competition and marketing, (5) human resources, (6) corporate structure, and (7) finance. Economic change is the focus of all seven areas, with trends and operational strategies outlined for hospitals, physicians, other providers (nursing homes, extended care facilities, and ambulatory care centers), and patients. Although practicing nurses were not included in the panels of experts who participated in the study, the document is well worth studying for implications for professional nursing.

Change Within Society

Nurses need now to look to the future and in doing so plan the destiny of the profession. Hallett, at the 1984 American Nurses' Association convention, spoke on how the economy of the post-industrial society will affect what is done, how it is done, and whether there is success or failure.[10] The biggest mistake society can make is to think it can continue as it is. Nursing will change—it will be what nurses make of it.

Naisbitt, looking at America today, has described areas of restructuring that are changing Americans' lives.[11]

The ten most important areas of restructuring, the megatrends, are:

1. the move from an industrial society to an information society,
2. the introduction of new technology into society creating a counterbalancing human response, "high touch,"

3. the world economy changing so that countries do not operate independently of one another, but in a global economic system,
4. the replacement of short-term planning with longer-term planning,
5. the decentralization of America,
6. the move from institutional dependence to self-reliance,
7. the shift from a representative democracy to a participatory democracy,
8. the replacement of hierarchies with a networking process,
9. the population movement in America from North and East to South and West,
10. the explosion of a multiple-option society.[12]

The move from an industrial society to an information society occurred in 1957 with the introduction of the telecommunication satellite.[13] In 1979, the number one occupation in the United States became clerk.[14] The second largest classification of workers is professional.[15] It is interesting that the role of the clinical nurse specialist was developed at the same time that the information society began.

The more technological America becomes, the more human response or "high touch" is needed for counter-balance. In hospitals, primary nursing is cited as an example of very high touch for patients.[16] Home care and birthing centers have become increasingly popular related to the human need for high touch.

The economy of America is moving from being national to global. All countries of the world are becoming interdependent as manufacturing becomes more competitive. The health care industry has become more global as information on available services in different parts of the world becomes known. Hospitals in the United States are marketing surgical services to all parts of the world. In a "package deal," patients are flown to the United States. Surgical services, as well as interpreters and family accommodations, are parts of the package. Patients from the United States are likewise traveling to foreign countries for medical services not yet available in the United States.

Long-term planning is replacing short-term planning for business and industry. Hospitals have developed long-range plans for the survival of the institutions. The hospital length of stay for patients has declined so that hospitals are developing marketing strategies and broadening services for the long-range institutional survival. Yet due to the economy and short-range planning, some hospitals will not survive.

With the decline of industry in America, centralization is moving to decentralization. Transition within nursing's professional organization, the American Nurses' Association, has moved into a federalist model. The local organization and particularly specialty groups are gaining strength at the expense of the national organization. Education for the master's degree prepared nurse has moved from a generalist education (administration, education) to a specialist education (clinical nurse specialist).

Americans are turning from institutional help to a self-help concept. The health care industry may feel the impact of the self-care concept more strongly than any other part of the society. People have reclaimed personal control over what happens to them in the areas of nutrition, hospices, home health care, natural child birth, holistic health, wellness programs, and the effects of the environment. There is a growing market for self-help kits. Americans can purchase, without medical advice, blood pressure testing apparatus, pregnancy test kits, materials for diabetes screening, and in a number of supermarkets and banks, automated sensors are available to check blood pressures and pulse rates for a nominal fee.

A shift of power has been occurring from a representative democracy to a participatory democracy. Americans are more interested in participating in events that affect them than they are in having someone represent them. In the 1980 elections, voters from four states, California, North Dakota, Missouri, and Michigan, cast more votes for initiatives and referenda than votes cast for governors.[17]

Initiatives brought about by voters have been issues on energy, the environment, and health. Banning herbicide spraying, requiring nonsmoking sections in business and public buildings, banning nonreturnable bottles and cans, limiting heights of newly constructed buildings, and attempting to prohibit nuclear power and the use of public funds for abortion are issues voters have recently decided upon.

Hierarchies are being replaced by the networking process. Networking is a means of communication in which the members treat one another as peers. It is the communication that creates a horizontal rather than a vertical link between people. Naisbitt states three reasons for the formation of networks: "the death of traditional structures, the din of information overload, and the past failure of hierarchies."[18] A health care institution that can develop a network style management system is creating an environment for collaborative practice. Nurses, physicians, dietitians, social workers, and consumers, by communicating across disciplines and with mutual respect, will have established a network and collaborative practice.

Population changes have and will continue to occur so that the southern and western areas of the United States are more populated than the northern and eastern. While the decline of industry and economy has occurred in the North and East, the industry and economy have increased in the South and West. For the health care industry, this megatrend should indicate where professional growth opportunities are most available.

The movement from an either/or to a multiple option society is most significant in the areas of the family and women. There is no one typical family of the 1980s. Families now include people living together not related by blood or marriage, single parent families, husband-wife households either with one working spouse or with both spouses working, and a greater number of people living alone. The value of the individual is increasing in today's society.

Women today have more options than ever before. Traditional roles for women have changed as a result of the women's movement and the changes in American families. Women can choose, as individuals, whether to work or not and are not bound by stereotyping of traditional women's work. Enrollment in nursing schools has declined, while one-third of students in medical schools are women.[19] More women are currently in college and graduate school programs than are men.[20] Randolph and Ross-Valliere state that the feminist movement has "rejected the nursing profession because of the female stereotype the profession portrays" and that "nursing, in turn, continues to isolate itself from the Women's Movement."[21] Some nurses perhaps never needed "liberation." There are nurses who were always career-oriented, made individual decisions about their own life styles, were assertive, and gained respect, support, and acceptance from peers and people in positions of power and authority.

All women have gained from the women's movement in areas of comparable worth, education, sexual stereotyping, establishing personal credit, and making decisions about their own life styles. Men have also gained from the women's movement. The number of men in nursing has increased, men are employed as secretaries, men are exercising their options to take maternity leave, and some men are full-time fathers while their spouses work.

THE FUTURE

Now, by looking at the environment, economics, current events, technology, consumers, and health care industry, the future for collaborative practice of the nursing profession can be examined. The environment of health care has and will continue to change from the hospital to the home or nursing home. As a result of the prospective payment system instituted by the federal government, patients are leaving hospitals sooner. Some of these patients are too ill to care for themselves at home. Others are so ill they are unable to return home until recuperation has occurred at the nursing home. With shorter lengths of stay, collaboration among consumers, physicians, and nurses must occur so that consumers' needs are met.

A true experience for one nurse and her neighbor provides an example of how collaboration or lack of collaboration can affect patients discharged from the hospital. The neighbor, a 70-year-old female with no relatives living locally, was discharged from a large medical center following an 18-day hospitalization. During the hospitalization, she was diagnosed as having diabetes mellitus, glomerulonephritis, septicemia, and extreme weakness in the upper right extremity, cause unknown. Hospital nurses had assisted the patient out of bed and for short walks down the corridor during the last four days of hospitalization. Upon discharge the patient was not only unable to walk alone but was too weak to move herself from a sitting or prone position to a standing position. The nurse-neighbor rented a walker on the day of discharge although no recommendation for such was made to the patient by the hospital staff. The nurse-neighbor was called on the telephone when the patient needed to change positions. The patient regained enough mobility within two days of discharge so that she could get up and down on her own.

Although the patient was discharged on seven different medications (including insulin), no medications or prescriptions were available to the patient upon hospital discharge. The patient was told by a hospital nurse to call the doctor for the prescriptions. At the insistence of the nurse-neighbor and against hospital policy, the patient was given the multiple-dose insulin vial the hospital nurses had been using in the hospital and several insulin syringes. Not until three days following discharge was the patient or the nurse-neighbor able to reach the private physician to obtain prescriptions for the seven discharge medications.

Dietary instructions were handed to the patient upon hospital discharge with the comment, "If you read this you will understand everything about your diet." For the 70-year-old patient that had never "dieted" in her life, this was far from true, and numerous learning sessions from the nurse-neighbor were required to achieve understanding.

Although the patient had been "instructed" on giving her own insulin injections, it was apparent to the nurse-neighbor that the patient could not read the numbers on the insulin syringe to draw up the correct dosage. A free-standing magnifying glass was purchased by the nurse-neighbor, and even with the upper right extremity weakness the patient was able to provide self-medication.

The patient expected that she was "ready" for discharge because the physician ordered it (she was happy to leave). The nurse-neighbor expected the patient to be discharged on self-care. The physician expected the patient to be "taught" by the time the patient was medically ready for discharge. The hospital nurses expected the patient to be readmitted soon after discharge due to lack of patient education related to diabetes management.

Collaboration among the consumer, physician, and nurses would have provided better care for this patient, and the expectations at discharge would have been more realistic.

Fortunately, this patient is doing remarkably well seven months after discharge and has not required further hospitalization. Had it not been for the nurse-neighbor providing home care and patient education, the outcome for this patient would be quite different. One can only speculate on the numbers of patients adversely affected by shorter lengths of stay and the lack of collaborative practice.

For patients going from hospital to home, private home health care agencies can provide much needed services, and these agencies will continue to grow. In 1980, 68 percent of hospitals in the United States were reportedly using primary nursing care.[22] The individualized care received, through the large extent that primary nursing care is practiced, needs to be incorporated into the home care patients receive. Primary nurses, collaborating with nurses in the home health care agencies, should increase and provide patients with an easier transition from hospital to home. This collaboration can provide more satisfaction to the consumer of services received during and after hospitalization.

Patients going from hospital to a nursing home, likewise, need the smooth transition that collaboration among nurses can provide. Nursing home nurses need more education on technical aspects of patient care. Nurses in the hospital and education settings can provide these services and create a networking resource for the nurses.

The high technology in the health care field is producing a field of moral technology. As organ transplants become more common, the area of medical-legal-moral issues becomes more important. Choices that have to be made can occur only with collaboration among nurses, physicians, consumers, and, at times, the government.

Consumers are wanting more control over the quality of their lives. Issues on whether to provide life support and for how long can be resolved only through collaboration of affected parties. Collaboration of affected parties must always include the consumer, the consumer's family, nurses, physicians, and others involved with the consumer's care. As the quality of life varies from individual to individual, so must the resolution of medical-legal-moral issues be individualized.

As society becomes more information-based, computers will be used in all aspects of health care. Hospitals currently use computers largely for tracking purposes: patients, supplies, and finances. Standards of nursing care will be computerized so that quality controls, costs, and reporting systems will be built into the programs. If the outcome of care has not been reached in a timely manner, the computer will notify the nurse. Collaboration among nurses is very important in establishing the standards and also in providing the high touch necessary for the information society.

Nurses, especially clinical nurse specialists, will have home computers that connect into hospital computers. The monitoring and progress of patient care will be determined and entered without leaving home. Collaboration with consumers and staff nurses will be of utmost importance in providing the high touch.

Collaborative research will be enhanced by the computer so that more nursing research will be collaborative. Collaborative nurse researchers will have access through the computer to data retrievals and analyses of their collaborators. Where population numbers available to one researcher are small, collaboration with other researchers having likewise small population numbers can provide significant studies in which the results can be generalized. Education programs are becoming available for nurses to learn computer usage and capabilities.

For the nurse executive, computer usage will be more like business usage today, with access to data from their office computers. Long-range effects of change can be predicted by using hypothetical and existing variables. The effects of an alternative care unit can be examined via the computer to determine the economic change to the institution, impact on staff, and usage by consumers. Ensuring that licensure for employed registered nurses is current can be tracked and annually updated by the computer. Nurse executives will need programs developed for their specific needs and programs developed in collaboration with other nurse executives. Computer programs needing development include studies to determine if the number of physicians' orders per patient affects the required hours of nursing care per patient; an objective patient classification system developed by computers tracking the ordering of patient supplies, medications, and the patient's length of stay; and programs to compare and contrast differences in nursing practices among units within the same institution and among units of different institutions.

More nurses, in the future, will be direct providers of health care and will receive direct reimbursement for services. Nurses will become involved in health maintenance, developing and being solely responsible for programs on stress reduction, weight reduction, and wellness programs. Consumers, either not able to pay the high costs charged by physicians or unwilling to pay the high costs, will turn to nurses for care. Consumers will find nurses as capable, more personable, and more cost efficient than physicians.

As more consumers demand these services, third party payers will allow this to occur. Some midwives currently practice independently of physicians, using physicians as consultants. Physicians are seeing midwifery practice as competitive to their own practice and oppose it. Nurses collaborating with consumers, physicians, and other nurses will convince physicians the change is good. Physicians will be providers of episodic illness care and surgical services, collaborating with the nurses in independent practice to provide post-hospital nursing care.

As budgets in hospitals and educational institutions become tighter, dual roles for nurses will increase. Nursing students will need education in settings outside the hospital as the hospital's patient population declines. Students will need to care for patients in the recuperative stage of illness to realize the outcome of nursing care provided in the acute or post-operative phase of illness. Dual roles will bring about increased collaboration between hospital and educational staffs. The base for this collaborative practice needs to be examined and perhaps negotiated. Time not spent with students or patients needs to be divided so that the administration's expectations for the educational institution are met as well as administration's expectations for the practice institution. Nurses cannot fulfill full-time expectations of both institutions.

Consumers of health care are examining options available to them and selecting from these options what will meet their individual needs. As nursing departments in hospitals individualize patient care through primary nursing, consumers will be better informed of the differences in nursing practices. Patients will learn that nursing care is what patients are admitted to hospitals for and that if medical care does not need the collaborative practice of nurses, medical care can be practiced on an outpatient basis. Self-care units will decline in number and usage, as consumers find health care that needs no nursing needs no hospitalization. Philadelphia's Presbyterian University, determining 10 percent of its patients could do without all the services and high technological equipment in the hospital, has opened a hotel/hospital across the street.[23] The private room charge for the hotel is $425 cheaper than the hospital room charge. The lengths of stay for hospitalized patients will be further reduced, and the collaboration of the consumer at home with the nurse in the hospital will be increased. Consumers in the hospital setting will be those patients acutely ill and recovering post-operatively. Consumer-nurse collaboration will occur, with nurses teaching consumers about post-discharge home care.

More nurses will need to practice in settings outside the hospital. All aspects of home care will grow so that the majority of nurses in practice will not be hospital-based. Nurses will be more flexible in their hours worked, as home care will expand from the current eight-to-five time period.

SUMMARY

Nurses need to evaluate their current practice, look at changes within the environment, economics, consumer expectations, technological advances, and health care practices to determine the direction of nursing practice. The professionalism of nursing can only occur within nursing. Nursing can no longer be reactionary to issues at hand but must make planned changes within nursing to move to a professional status. An attribute of professionalism (as discussed in Chapter 4) is control over practice, so that for nursing to move forward professionally, nurses have to change nursing. These changes can occur only through nurse-to-nurse collaboration.

NOTES

1. A. Merriam Webster, *Webster's New Collegiate Dictionary* (Springfield, Mass.: G.C. Merriam Co., 1974), pp. 185–186.

2. Ingeborg G. Mauksch and Mary H. Miller, *Implementing Change in Nursing* (St. Louis, Mo.: C.V. Mosby Co., 1981), p. 9.

3. Kurt Lewin, *Field Theory in Social Science: Selected Theoretical Papers,* ed. Dorwin Cartwright (New York: Harper & Row, Publishers, 1951), pp. 19–23.

4. Ibid., pp. 24–39.

5. Kurt Lewin, "Group Decision and Social Change," in *Readings in Social Psychology,* ed. T.M. Newcomb and E.L. Hartley (New York: Holt, Rinehart and Winston, 1958), pp. 207–209.

6. Grace L. Deloughery, *History and Trends of Professional Nursing,* 8th ed. (St. Louis, Mo.: C.V. Mosby Co., 1977), pp. 153–154.

7. Mark Vogel, "The Transformation of the American Hospital, 1850–1920," in *Health Care in America: Essays in Social History,* ed. Susan Reverby and David Rosner (Philadelphia: Temple University Press, 1979), pp. 162–185.

8. Franklin A. Shaffer, "Prospective Payment: A Strategic Plan for Nursing Power," in *Power Politics and Policy In Nursing,* ed. Rita Reis Wieczorek (New York: Springer Publishing Company, 1985), pp. 33–38.

9. Arthur Anderson and Company, *Health Care In The 1990's: Trends and Strategies* (Chicago, Ill.: Arthur Anderson and Company and The American College of Hospital Administrators, 1984), pp. 1–2.

10. Jeffrey Hallet, *The New Economy* (Presentation at the American Nurses' Association Convention, New Orleans, June 1984).

11. John Naisbitt, *Megatrends* (New York: Warner Books, Inc., 1982), pp. 1–2.

12. Ibid., pp. 12, 39, 55, 79, 97, 131, 159, 189, 207, 231.

13. Ibid., pp. 11–12.

14. Ibid., p. 14.

15. Ibid., p. 15.

16. Ibid., p. 42.

17. Ibid., p. 166.

18. Ibid., p. 197.

19. John E. Skandalakis, "The Future of Nursing: Some Facts, Opportunities, and Challenges to Consider," *Journal of the Medical Association of Georgia* 71, no. 10 (1982): 711–713.

20. John Naisbitt, *Megatrends* (New York: Warner Books, Inc., 1982), p. 235.

21. Bonnie Moore Randolph and Clydene Ross-Valliere, "Consciousness Raising Groups," *The American Journal of Nursing* 79, no. 5 (1979): 922.

22. Karen L. Ciske, "Will Primary Nursing Survive in the 80's?," *Nursing Administration Quarterly* 5, no. 3 (1981): 79–80.

23. "Trends," *Forbes* 135, no. 5 (1985): 10.

SUGGESTED READINGS

Abdellah, F.G. "Future Directions of the Profession." *Imprint* 30, no. 2 (1983): 91, 93–94, 97.

Bishop, J.K. "Leadership and the Political Change Process." *Topics in Clinical Nursing* 6, no. 1 (1984): 10–16.

Elliott, J.E., and Osgood, G.A. "Federal Nursing Priorities for the 1980's." In *Nursing in the 1980's: Crises, Opportunities, Challenges.* Ed. L.H. Aiken and S.R. Gortner. Philadelphia: J.B. Lippincott Co., 1982, pp. 451–457.

Kemp, V.H. "An Overview of Change and Leadership." *Topics in Clinical Nursing* 6, no. 1 (1984): 1–9.

Leininger, M. "Futurology of Nursing: Goals and Challenges for Tomorrow." In *The Nursing Profession: Views Through the Mist.* Ed. N.L. Chaska. New York: McGraw-Hill Book Company, 1978, pp. 379–396.

Mauger, B.L., and Huggins, K. "Developing and Implementing Collaborative Nursing Education Research in the South." *Nursing Research* 29, no. 3 (1980): 189–192.

Mauksch, I.G. "Nursing in the 80's: The Critical Issues." *Arizona Nurse* 36, no. 1 (1983): 5–16.

Padilla, G.V., and Padilla G.J., "Nursing Roles to Improve Patient Care." *Nursing Digest,* Winter 1979, pp. 1–13.

Schlotfeldt, R.M. "The Nursing Profession: Vision of the Future." In *The Nursing Profession: Views Through the Mist.* Ed. N.L. Chaska. New York: McGraw-Hill Book Company, 1978, pp. 397–404(a).

Schlotfeldt, R.M. "Nursing in the Future." *Nursing Outlook* 29, no. 5 (1981): 295–301(b).

Sheridan, D.R. "The Health Care Industry in the Marketplace: Implications for Nursing." *The Journal of Nursing Administration* 3, no. 9 (1983): 36–40.

Styles, M.M. "The Vision." *On Nursing Toward a New Endowment.* St. Louis, Mo.: C.V. Mosby Co., 1982, pp. 229–234.

Index

About the Contributors

Joyce Patricia Brockhaus, R.N., M.S.N., Ph.D. Dr. Brockhaus is a Clinical Nurse Specialist in child psychiatry at St. Louis Children's Hospital and clinical faculty member in the Department of Child Psychiatry at Washington University School of Medicine. She maintains a private practice in child and family counseling specializing in the area of adoption.

Her previous work experience includes teaching in and coordinating graduate programs in psychiatric/mental health nursing as well as working as a staff nurse in a residential treatment center for emotionally disturbed children. She is listed in *Who's Who in the Midwest* and *Notable Americans*. Her areas of writing include adoption, values clarification, adolescents, and stress management. Dr. Brockhaus's writings have appeared in both scholarly journals and textbooks.

Linda S. Cape, R.N., M.S.N. Linda Cape received her B.S.N. from the University of Kansas, Lawrence, Kansas in 1973 and her M.S.N. from St. Louis University, St. Louis, Missouri in 1979. She is currently a clinical nurse specialist in neonatology at St. Louis Children's Hospital and has functioned in that capacity since 1979. She has presented numerous papers, co-edited the book *Coping with Caring for Sick Newborns,* W.B. Saunders, 1982, and co-authored a chapter in *Persuading Physicians,* Aspen Systems Corp., 1984.

Doris Asselmeier England, R.N., M.S.N., F.A.A.N. Doris England has been employed at St. Louis Children's Hospital since 1965. She has served as Director of Nursing Service, Director of Patient Care, and currently is Vice President, Patient Care. In this capacity she serves as the administrator for numerous hospital departments including nursing, pharmacy, social service, respiratory care, and risk management.

Doris England is active in professional and community groups and has served as President of the American Society for Nursing Service Administrators, Chairman of the Council on Nursing of the American Hospital Association, President of the University of Missouri Alumni Association, and Board Member of Edgewood Children's Home. She is a Fellow in the American Academy of Nursing, a member of Sigma Theta Tau, and is the recipient of the alumni award from the University of Missouri as well as the citation of merit from the School of Nursing of the University of Missouri-Columbia.

Audrey Kalafatich, R.N., Ed.D., F.A.A.N. Dr. Kalafatich has been an educator in various institutions across the country, holding the rank of full professor in her last university position. While teaching she also participated in clinical practice both in hospitals and in a teenage clinic setting. Currently, she is a Clinical Nurse Specialist, Adolescent Care, at St. Louis Children's Hospital; is Chairperson of the Committee for Nursing Research; and is currently engaged in her own research on stress and coping in hospitalized teenagers.

Amy Hemme Kennedy, R.N., M.S.N. Amy Kennedy is a Clinical Specialist in Nursing of Children at St. Louis Children's Hospital. She received her B.S.N. from the University of Missouri, Columbia, Missouri, and her M.S.N. from St. Louis University, St. Louis, Missouri.

She has been a Clinical Specialist in Nursing of Children for 12 years with experience in birth defects, cystic fibrosis, nephrology, and general pediatrics. Her special interests are: chronic illness in pediatric patients, family centered care, motivation of nursing personnel, primary nursing, and community education for pediatric nursing.

Carol Hill Luckey, R.N., M.S.N. (R). Carol Hill Luckey is currently a Clinical Nurse Specialist at St. Louis Children's Hospital working with pediatric medical patients and is a project director for a special nursing research grant from the Department of Health and Human Services. Ms. Luckey is a graduate of Barnes Hospital School of Nursing and has completed requirements for the degrees of Bachelor of Science in Nursing and Masters of Science in Nursing (Research) at St. Louis University. She has held positions of staff nurse, head nurse, supervisor, and patient care consultant at St. Louis Children's Hospital.

Bobbie J. Mackay, R.N., M.S.N., M.S.W. Bobbie J. Mackay is currently a Clinical Nurse Specialist at St. Louis Children's Hospital working with children with chronic lung disease. In addition, she coordinates the hospital-wide patient/family education program. Ms. Mackay is a graduate of the School of Nursing at the University of South Carolina where she received a Bachelor of Science degree. She completed the requirements for Masters of Science degree in Nursing of Children at St. Louis University in 1975. She has held a variety of positions throughout her nursing career: staff nurse in a pediatric intensive care unit and in a pediatric psychiatric and drug treatment center; clinical instructor at St. Louis University School of Nursing; seminar instructor for a chronic illness course at St. Louis University School of Nursing; and clinical specialist at St. Louis Children's Hospital.

Robin Moushey, R.N., M.S.N. Robin Moushey graduated from Barnes School of Nursing with a diploma in 1968. She received her B.S.N. in 1974 from St. Louis University and her M.S.N. from St. Louis University in 1977. Her previous positions include: staff nursing, infection control nurse, clinical instructor in diploma and baccalaureate programs, and staff development instructor.

In her current position as Clinical Nurse Specialist for General Surgery, job responsibilities include coordination of care of children undergoing surgery. Specific groups of children are those infants and children with gastrointestinal conditions, children who are burned or have been in major accidents, children with abdominal tumors, and all children with Broviac catheters.

Mary Mills Redman, R.N., M.S.N. Ms. Redman completed her B.S.N. at Vanderbilt University and her M.S.N. at St. Louis University. She is currently a Ph.D. candidate in the area of counselor education at St. Louis University. As a Clinical Specialist in Neurology and Neurosurgery at St. Louis Children's Hospital, her current position includes responsibility for patient care, education, consultation, and research and publication in the field of her specialization.

Anne T. Richardson, R.N., M.S.N. Anne T. Richardson received her R.N. and B.S.N. from Vanderbilt University School of Nursing (1966) and her M.S.N. in the Nursing of Children from St. Louis University School of Nursing (1976). She has been an active nurse for the entire period including 3 years of staff and office experience, 7 years as a nurse educator, and the remainder as a Clinical Nurse Specialist. The vast majority of her experience has been in the area of nursing of children and families. Her clinical expertise is applied mainly toward clients experiencing a variety of levels of renal involvement.

Valann Tasch, R.N., M.S.N., C.P.N.P. Valann Tasch received her diploma from St. John's Nursing School, St. Louis, Missouri and her B.S.N. from Washington University, St. Louis, Missouri. She received her Master's Degree from the University of Wisconsin at Madison in Nursing Care of Children. She attended the Washington University School of Medicine Pediatric Nurse Practitioner program and was certified in 1978. She has worked in the inpatient hospital setting as a Clinical Nurse Specialist in General Pediatrics and most recently as a Clinical Nurse Specialist/Pediatric Nurse Practitioner in outpatient Neurology where she provides services to clients with neurological problems and their families.